The Energetic

Anatomy of a Yogi

- Healing the Emotional and Mental Body through Yoga -

by Paul G. Balch and Jaylee Balch

Strategic Book Publishing and Rights Co.

Paul and Jaylee Balch wish to acknowledge the following people:

The late Patrick Desplace—for being a brilliant teacher and mentor who laid the foundational knowledge for our healing path.

The late Ciril—for being the Master of Masters and for his seen and unseen guidance on every level, always.

Mr. Lui, the Tao Master—for making all the difference with his love and patience.

Jonny Mauk—for his extreme postures on the Flat Irons, Colorado.

This is for all the yoga studios who gave us the opportunity to host the Seminar.

Last but not least, the tens of thousands who crossed our path over twenty-five years— you were our teachers, too.

If it were not for Paul B. and his amazing ability to hold all this knowledge in his consciousness, the book would not be possible! Love, light & Laughter Jaylee B.

"Our deepest fear is not that we are inadequate.
Our deepest fear is that we are powerful beyond measure.
It is our light, not our darkness that most frightens us."
—Nelson Mandela

Strategic Book Publishing and Rights Co.
12620 FM 1960, Suite A4-507
Houston TX 77065
www.sbpra.com

ISBN: 978-1-62212-350-6

Contents

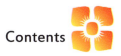

I Am the greatest love story by Jaylee Balch

Part One: Personal Information and Previews   1
About the Authors   2
Foreword by the Authors   5
Declaration by the Authors   6
A Review of "Anatomy of a Yogi" Seminar   8
Yoga is Yoga is Yoga   10

Part Two: The Mind & the Inner Self   13
Energy and Healing   14
Living in Touch with Nature   16
Meditation, Contemplation & Concentration   17
The Five Minds   19
Free Will   22
Going Beyond Past Patterns   22

Part Three: The Chakra systam   25
Introduction to the Seven Main Chakras   26
Chakra Secret   26
Corresponding Chakras in Limbs and Torso   27
Explanation on the Three Chakra Layers   32
Kundalini Chakra   33
Sacral Chakra   35
Solar Plexus Chakra   37
Heart Chakra   39
Throat Chakra   41
Forehead Chakra   43
Crown Chakra   45
The Emotional Organs   46
The Two Sides for Your Body   48
The Celestial Symphony: Poem   50

Part Four: The Energetics of Postures   51
FEAR   52
Awkward Pose   53
Balancing Stick Pose   57
Boat (Sit-up) Pose   60
PEOPLE   62
Breath of Fire Pose   64
Bridge Pose   65
Camel Pose   67
Cobblers Pose   69
Cobra Pose   71

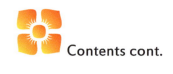

Contents cont.

STRESS	74
Crescent Lunge/Warrior Pose	76
Dancers Pose	78
Dead Body Pose	81
BELIEFS	82
Deep Breathing Pose	84
Downward Facing Dog Pose	86
TIME MANAGEMENT	88
Eagle Pose	90
Fixed Firm Pose	93
Frog Pose	95
Full Locust Pose	97
REACTIONS	98
Floor Bow/Wheel Pose	100
Gorilla Pose	102
Half Moon Pose	104
Half Pigeon Pose	106
INTUITION	108
Half Spine Twist Pose	110
Half Tortoise Pose	112
Head to Knee with Stretching Pose	114
I want to play with the gods: Poem	117
CHOICE	118
Headstand Pose	120
Locust Pose	122
Rabbit Pose	124
LOVE	126
Shoulder Stand Pose	128
Standing Forehead to Knee Pose	130
Standing Separate Leg Stretching Pose	132
CHANGE	134
Standing Separate Leg Head to Knee Pose	136
Tree Pose	138
Toe Stand Pose	140
Ever Wonder Who Held the Pen?: Poem	141
MAGNETISM	142
Triangle Pose	144
Wind Removing Pose	146
BE MINDFUL	148
References	150

I AM the greatest love story

From when time began and even before, I loved you.
I loved you from the rising of the sun to the setting of its glow.
As My fingers reached on the rays and touched mankind
So I marvelled at the sight of what I had created.
From the flicker of a leaf in the August wind
I learnt to understand your sensitivity
From the cry of a triumphant eagle
I learnt your freedom and what it was worth
From the bold dash of a frightened mouse
I learnt of your vulnerability and its fear
From the boastful roar of the majestic lion
I learnt your pride and your sense of survival
From the pack of wild dogs and hyenas
I learnt your cunning and your unity
From the snake, so clever and fearless
I learnt your solitude and your power
From the hummingbird, so miniscule
I learnt your intentions and courage
From the giraffe, tall and peaceful
I learnt your grace and compassion for all
From the magnificent beast, the elephant
I learnt to measure your protectiveness
From the swaying of the summer papyrus
I learnt your moods and their various ways
From the stars that abide in the heavens
I learnt your brightness and tenacity
From the rolling of a boulder over sands
I learnt your determination and willpower
From the last snowflake of a cold winter
I learnt your uniqueness and design
From the moon and its changing form
I learnt your gifts and your seasons
From the spring of every new year
I learnt of your renewed unfoldment
From the last breath of a full life
I learnt that you loved Me, only Me
From all of these above and so much more
I learnt that I AM the greatest love story.

—Jaylee Balch

PART ONE: PERSONAL INFORMATION AND PREVIEWS

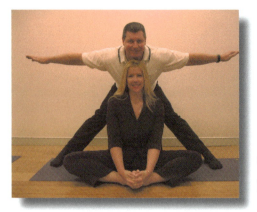

About Paul G Balch

Paul Balch grew up in a family that played state-level sports, including rugby, squash, and boxing. As a young adult growing up in Darwin, Australia, he did a building apprenticeship and spent years in the medical field. His ability to fine tune his natural sensitivity developed during long hours hurrying around hospitals and tending to sick people. Like many in his profession, he was initiated into the catastrophes and small hours of the graveyard shift. In his experiences working with people in hospital, he developed a curiosity to know more and learn more about the human phenomenon.

For his whole life, he has wanted to know the secrets. He has wanted to know about the afterlife and where emotions are channelled once they are felt and what their purposes are. In a series of bursts over fifteen years, he studied massage, anatomy and physiology, relaxation, hypnotherapy, psychology, meditation, energy healing, reiki, dreams, tarot, astral projection, and alchemy, an eclectic combination of tools he would come to treasure in later years. Perhaps the most impacting experience that was carved into his path was a death experience he had while in the remote Australian bush. From that point on, he met, studied, and worked with a master of the development of human potential for twenty years. It was in these years that he got to meet a Tibetan Lama, a being

IF MAN DOES NOT KNOW WHO BREATHES WITHIN HIM AND IF MAN DOES NOT KNOW WHO DREAMS WITHIN HIM, IT IS NOT BECAUSE THERE IS ONE SELF WHO ACTS IN THE PHYSICAL UNIVERSE AND ANOTHER WHO DREAMS AND BREATHES. IT IS BECAUSE HE HAS BURIED THE PART OF HIMSELF WHICH BREATHES AND DREAMS.
- UNKNOWN -

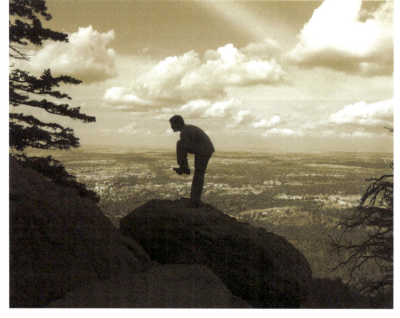

ENTERING STILLNESS - JONNY MAUK - BIKRAM YOGA WORLD CHAMPION

of indescribable magnitude and knowingness who currently mentors Paul as he teaches worldwide.

In the '90s, he was introduced to yoga and was instantly attracted to its gains and benefits and how he could apply his knowledge to the yogic world. Paul has facilitated over 10,000 one-on-one coaching / self development sessions with clients resulting in life changing benefits ranging from subtle lifestyle adjustments to significant transformational achievements on both a professional and personal level.

Having worked with energy and emotional aspects of people's bodies over many years, Paul could see many aspects of yoga that could be enhanced to transform, heal, and empower people even more. In the early 2000s he met his wife and teaching partner, Jaylee, and together they travel for most of the year, bringing awareness to the human spirit and awakening in individuals their true potential through various modalities including their sequence of Sundara Jiva Yoga©.

About Jaylee Balch

Jaylee was inspired twenty years ago to pursue a path of self development and to discover the depth of human affairs. Having completed a double Bachelor of Art Degree in

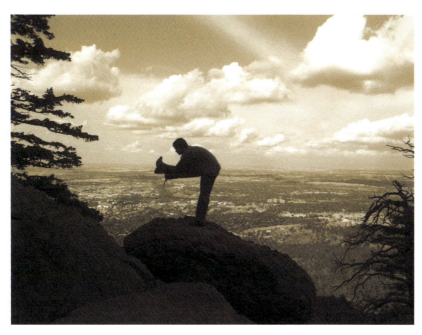

KNOWING STILLNESS - JONNY MAUK - BIKRAM YOGA WORLD CHAMPION

Psychology and Communications, she challenged herself in the field of Marketing by pursuing a career in a Design House where she was responsible for the corporate image of over 100 companies in South Africa. Jaylee worked extensively in publishing, editing and media relations. After a number of years, Jaylee expanded her career to include public relations where she was responsible for designing, coordinating and executing some of the largest events in the African Hospitality and Entertainment Industry. Gaining diverse experience, she successfully worked with an extensive group of multicultural clientele. Working in these industries highlighted a need for managing the stress within the business environment, while balancing the creative edge. This then motivated Jaylee to pursue a new career path in life coaching.

Over the past seven years Jaylee has been lecturing and coaching individuals in stress management and personal development around the world. Jaylee is an inspirational speaker with expertise including, leadership and transformation of individuals and teams, empowering small to medium sized businesses, motivational speaking focused on achieving excellence, and helping women realise their full potential in their work and personal lives. Augmenting her pursuit of group and individual growth, Jaylee is focused upon developing programs empowering people to create more effectively and develop lateral thinking. With two books in publishing, she is currently running workshops across three continents and has built a global network of clients within the retail, cosmetic, health, telecommuni-

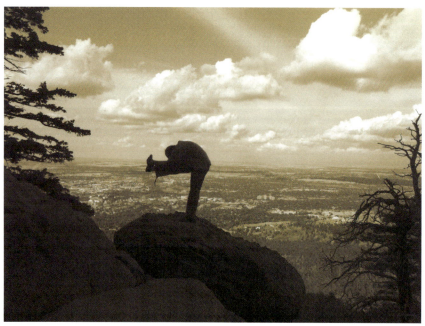

MASTERING STILLNESS - JONNY MAUK - BIKRAM YOGA WORLD CHAMPION

cations, medical, information technology and recruitment industries. She currently holds a Hatha Yoga Teaching Certification to add to her skills.

As a Hypnotherapist she focusses on her studies and experiences in her world, to combines much of the spiritual and emotional content into seminars and helps people uncover blockages and find emotional freedom.

She had the fortune to meet and be initiated into the Tao and Tibetan lineages under their respective Masters and is currently mentored by them. She combines her talents with Paul's in their focus to empower people and bring healing to those who need it. Having spent years as a professional graphic designer, she used her talent to design this book for the world to see. As a photographer, the pictures in each drawing are from her own collection.

It is important to note that they both work intensely with the Toltec tradition, Lazaris, Kryon, Tao tradition, Ancient Mystery Schools, and Tibetan tradition.

Foreword by the Authors

We believe and know yoga to be a spiritual practice and in the west we have reduced that to being a purely physical practice in many areas. We do understand that even the practice of the asana (physical postures) is of great benefit to many, although many are too busy or don't understand the spiritual side of it. We believe the purpose of yoga is to unite the mind, the body, and the spirit to bring each person closer to inner peace and self-awareness. We question each person's need to exercise the physical body without thought or with neglect of the emotional, mental, and spiritual bodies. It is essential for us to be healthy and whole and exercise all aspects of our being, and if we neglect one aspect imbalances occur, which left unresolved eventually manifest disease.

So the motivation and purpose for Sundara Jiva Yoga© is to take the practice of the asana to a whole new level of experience, awareness, healing, and creativity, understanding the energetic and emotional aspects of the body and bringing in the spiritual side of your practice. Our purpose of creating Sundara Jiva Yoga© is to empower yogis and yoginis to a level where they can self-diagnose and release their own emotional and energetic blocks and eventually harness their natural energy flow to be more creative. Through this book and practice you will learn how to scan your physical body and understand where your blocks are and what you are releasing and healing. This takes your yoga healing to a conscious emotional and mental level where you can understand the blocks and the causes

WHERE SHOULD YOU BE? ...EXACTLY WHERE YOU ARE RIGHT NOW. WHAT SHOULD YOU BE DOING? ...EXACTLY WHAT YOU ARE DOING.

behind the blocks. A word on what we have found with many practitioners of yoga is the trap of becoming too involved with your body and being controlled by how your body feels or looks and functions. As a spiritual process you need to be in touch with and respect the physical level, which relates to your body and your environment, but not obsessed and controlled by it. Many people are off in a daydream hoping life was different, and others are so controlled by the physical (including materialism) that they are oblivious to anything more in life. This creates imbalances, so the purpose of Sundara Jiva Yoga© is to balance these aspects and to awaken and integrate all aspects of your being. Get ready to enjoy the ride for life through the Sundara Jiva Yoga© Experience.

Declaration by the Authors

Although Anatomy of a Yogi is a self-observation process, it is not the intent of the authors to diagnose any ailments and injuries. That is solely reserved for qualified medical people. They merely offer another perspective in dealing with the energetic and emotional healing of the body. They do not recommend that you stop any medication nor ignore the advice of your doctor or therapist but simply use the yoga postures to improve your quality of life. Yes, people have given up medicines after healing through yoga and have had physical injuries completely healed, but you need to work with your body holistically. There have been startling results and shifts in ailments and injuries; however, the degree of healing is personal and different for each person. With persistence, healing is possible, and if the practitioner follows the direction of the yoga teacher, there is no doubt that change for the better will occur.

At best, read the book and allow yourself to be open to what you read within and give those words that touch your heart a moment. Allow yourself to be honest, keeping your peace and knowing that just your contemplation of an energy allows it to change. Most of the energy blocks in the Energtic Anatomy of a Yogi don't even occur to the average person, but once you have read of them, you can self-examine your own life. No one has to know what blockages you discover. What you share is up to you. However, by simply doing the postures with those particular blocked emotions in mind you will begin a change of effect that with persistence could change your life completely.

Each posture is aligned with chakras and you will see some overlapping or similar characteristics throughout the book. No posture is completely the same as another so feel which one has the exact energy that you require to be released. You will begin to get a sense of how the energies work with the chakras and you will also notice that many postures deal with sexual issues. Simply, look at the use of ankles, wrists, sacral chakra, and pelvis and you will know why. As many postures require bending or pelvic work, sexuality is a big part of dealing with issues. Whether it is a backbend or a forward bend, the sacral chakra is being engaged.

For many people, sexuality is a difficult subject to broach and many don't even want to consider half the issues related to it. We suggest that you read with an open mind, consider yourself (privately), and allow yourself to be honest. Honesty does not cost anything. If you discover a sexual block, simply do the pose with the intent to release the block and watch what happens. As with everything, if a block has been lodged for many years, perhaps an ongoing yoga practice is needed . . . perhaps a few.

Each person is different!

Approach every class with a fresh mind and how you walk into the class will affect the quality of class that you have. Go in with a sense of humour because there will be that posture you don't get right or balance that keeps failing you. Remember: Your right side is masculine and your left side feminine; therefore, look at your balance. Which side do you fall out and which side is stronger? These are all clues to reading your body and where you need to work some issues out. Where is your body tight or stiff and which chakra does that relate to? Which side is weaker and where do you fall out of postures? Ask these questions and observe your yoga practice until you really get to know yourself.

Remember: Each body is different; therefore, the person next to you may do a posture deeper or hold it longer. Have respect for how you are built and how you work with your body. If you are double jointed, know your limits and engage those muscles to protect your joints. If you are flexible, work on strength and balance. Above all, focus and keep the mind quiet and don't allow the monkey mind to control you through your class. You walk the dog; the dog does not walk you. It is your class. Forget anyone exists and do the work to heal yourself and enjoy the journey! Follow the teacher and be conscious of your body as you listen, observe, feel, and release.

Enjoy yoga!

YOU CAN'T CHANGE YOUR GENES. THEY AREN'T IN CHARGE. WHAT CONTROLS YOUR BODY IS HOW YOUR CELLS PERCEIVE YOUR ENVIRONMENT. WHAT CONTROLS YOUR CELLS' PERCEPTIONS IS YOUR BELIEFS.
- DR BRUCE LIPTON -

A Review of "Anatomy of a Yogi" Seminar

by an independant source -

A Review of the "Anatomy of a Yogi" To all yoga practitioners, yoga is a window that allows us to glimpse into ourselves and to better understand our inner workings—physical, mental, and spiritual—and how these are affected by the world around us. This is the case, whether at a conscious or subconscious level. Have you ever wondered why some days you may find your practice ever-consuming while others you outshine your expectations? On occasion, do you find certain emotions, feelings, and/or memories arising during or after carrying out a particular posture or during final Savasana? Perhaps you've wanted to unlock the mysteries of why you favour some postures while you anticipate others with reluctance.

In the yoga studios' continued dedication to yoga practitioners, to use yoga as a means to better understand ourselves, on Sunday, June 3, 2007, Paul and Jaylee Balch were invited to hold an all-day seminar titled "Anatomy of a Yogi," which addressed these and many similar questions. The seminar was a resounding success with a number of participants who were presented with a comprehensive, detailed, and eloquent presentation that related the chakra system to emotional energetics; in particular as these relate to the postures in hot yoga practice.

Jaylee's skills as a graphic artist opportunely provided for the remarkable slide presentation that accompanied the seminar, with an abbreviated version of the slides provided to participants in a very useful and insightful hand-out, which can be regularly consulted for discerning answers to enquiries on the mind-body connection, specifically relating to the twenty-six postures.

Paul and Jaylee described emotions as "energy in motion." These are influenced by our perceptions of the past, present, and future. Past experiences result in hardwiring in the hindbrain. These become our reference points for expectations of what is occurring in the present or what is yet to come in the future. In life, this may translate to a person making a statement that he/she always attracts negative people into his/her life, and having this become a self-fulfilling prophecy. In yoga practice, it may be your expectations of how you will perform in a given posture, in light of previous practices. The present moment, on the other hand, draws on the powers of the frontal brain. This is where you can exercise free will and choice. Though it may be intermingled with the hardwiring of the hindbrain and reference points in the past, it has the potential for limitless possibilities in light of the boundless promises of the future. In the microcosm of yoga practice and in the macrocosm of life, it translates to letting go of expectations and, with each opportunity, welcoming what may, realizing the infinite prospects that lie ahead.

According to Paul and Jaylee, the unexpressed emotions—whether anger, sadness, love, or joy—become trapped within the body. Given the chakra system, which according to the yoga philosophy consists of spinning wheels of energy residing in various centres of the body, these trapped emotions will settle into various body parts suitable to the interactions of the energetics of the chakras to which the emotions connect. Consequently, you can use your yoga practice as an interface between your mind and body. As the body parts are flexed, twisted, compressed, and stretched, the emotional components released will manifest themselves. If you tap into these emerging patterns, you begin the dialogue between your mind and body. You can therefore use your hot yoga practice as a means to emotional healing. You may even more proactively set intentions towards this healing through your yoga. Given the limited scope of this article relative to the extensive amount of information covered by Paul and Jaylee in a full-day seminar, an attempt to summarize their vast captivating presentation may be futile and may do it disservice. It's best to get a glimpse by illustrating with one example.

The start of the series, Pranayama Breathing, provides an appropriate instance. On the surface, it clearly exercises the respiratory, circulatory, and nervous systems. But beyond the obvious, given its emphasis on the neck, shoulders, and chest (which connect with the fourth and fifth chakras), subtle interactions of the fourth and fifth—the heart and throat—chakras result in its effect on emotional energetics associated with these chakras. The neck is a body part vital in its association with decision-making, as is exemplified by the expression "sticking one's neck out" for a cause. By exercising the neck, you therefore begin the yoga sequence with moving forward, not holding back with indecision. The shoulders are an expression towards the surrounding environment and external obligations, as noted in the phrase "carrying a burden on one's shoulders."

Thus, you commence the series by releasing said obligations and focusing on yourself. The heart relates with matters of intimacy and love; hence, according to Paul and Jaylee's interpretation, the breathing helps with delivery of "unexpressed emotions towards inti-

YOUR NATURAL STATE IS JOY, LOVE AND ABUNDANCE IN EVERYTHING. EVERYTHING ELSE IS ARTIFICIAL AND AN ERROR
- BARBARA MOHR -

mate ones and fear of being oneself." To more specifically apply these concepts, as a case in point, perhaps experiencing neck pain would convey the likelihood of indecision with regards to a particular choice in life.

In addition to discussing the twenty-six postures in detail within this framework, Paul and Jaylee presented participants with various meditation exercises that could be performed on a regular basis outside of the yoga studio to utilize and improve mental focus and concentration. Finally, the lecture portion was followed by a yoga class taught by Paul himself, which set the information into context for the attendees. The learning experience was one of enlightenment, clarifications, and many epiphanies, taking the awareness of the participants to new levels concerning emotional anatomy, thoughts, and attitudes as they apply to yoga more generally to life.

— by Roxana Mavai

Yoga is Yoga is Yoga

I can't remember when I first started doing hot yoga. Maybe 2001? I've never been a dedicated practitioner, often due to there being no studio in my town, or teaching so much that I didn't have time to go to classes and do a home practice. But I've done quite a bit of yoga over the years. Enough to know that if yoga were just about the physical, that I should be nice and bendy by now. I mean, how long does it take to lengthen a hamstring? Or release the hips? A year or so ago, I was fortunate enough to attend a Hot Yoga workshop by Paul and Jaylee Balch called "Anatomy of a Yogi." Paul is a trained Bikram and Hatha yoga teacher, but he's been studying all manner of spiritual ways, paths, texts, and teachings for something like three decades, much of it with masters of various stripes.

In this workshop, he and Jaylee go in depth into each posture and what's really going on when we practice Hot Yoga from a physical, mental, emotional, and spiritual perspective. Because while many styles of Hot Yoga may be primarily taught as a physical style of yoga stripped and devoid of all spiritual and philosophic undertones, you can't strip out its energetic effect no matter how you teach it. Whether people realise it or not, practicing Hot Yoga is going to affect them emotionally, mentally, and spiritually. And people doing yoga start to transform, whether they like it or not. Physically, mentally, emotionally, and even spiritually. But sometimes we don't transform physically as fast we as think we should. I've been practicing yoga of all stripes pretty damn steadily for ten years or more, yet still struggle to straighten my legs, and I wanted to know: What the hell am I holding on to so tightly that's preventing my hamstrings from softening and releasing like well-chewed gum?

I found out during the "Anatomy of a Yogi" workshop. See, according the way Paul and Jaylee see the world, we haven't just got one body. We've got four. There's the physical, emotional, mental, and spiritual bodies. And emotions? Think of them like energy in motion, felt sensations in the body that move. Except when we repress them, ignore them, or deny them, which is pretty much all of the time in today's world, that energy in motion gets stuck in the physical body because it has to go somewhere . . .

Same kind of thing with thoughts, beliefs, ideas, our concept of self, identity, the way things should be . . . this also gets stuck in the mental body. All of this—things stuck in the emotional and mental body—eventually show up in the physical body: in the way we manifest ourselves, in the ways we move, where we're tight, where we're weak. I've known this for a long time, simply because when I practiced yoga the movement of asana made me feel things. Hot Yoga in particular would trigger oceans of tears that would start in Dancer's Pose and continue for the whole damn series.

For a long time I wondered, why Dancer's? What was it about that posture that made me feel all these tears? During that workshop, I found out, and boy did it make sense. I also found out why my hamstrings have been tight, why my cobra has sucked lately, and what's been up with everything from Toe-Stand to Floor Bow. Each day of the workshop, Paul and Jaylee took us through the postures in detail and looked at which chakras were affected and what type of emotional and mental holding patterns had the opportunity to be released. Things like self-sabotage (who knew?), self-pity, forgiveness, integration of public and private self, opening to giving and receiving, letting go of resentment towards men and towards women. On and on it went . . . and as I listened I found I was developing a new appreciation for the elegance and the magic of the Hot Yoga series.

After each afternoon of lectures, we then got a chance to apply our newly learned (or validated!) knowledge to a class. It was such a sublime experience to be lead through the series with the usual Hot Yoga dialogue plus a whole series of new cues reminding us of what emotional or mental patterns we could release in this pose. Just knowing what the

11

potential blocks could be in each pose meant I could discern how to work within the pose—when to surrender, when to soften, when to strengthen, when to hold, when to be. Poses that had felt locked for the longest time were suddenly accessible. As a result of the workshop, my whole relationship to Hot Yoga changed.

Hot Yoga is as powerful a yoga practice as we make it—it's as powerful and as spiritual as our relationship with it. If we practice with awareness of the emotional, mental, and spiritual bodies—as well as the physical—then Hot Yoga will transform us on the path of self-realisation just like any other practice. It may not be for everyone, but it's definitely for some of us.

— by Kara-Leah Grant

(Kara-Leah Grant is a born and bred Kiwi girl. She publishes, edits, and otherwise nurtures New Zealand's own kick-arse yoga website, The Yoga Lunchbox, on a mission to make yoga a part of daily life in New Zealand.)

Part Two: The Mind & the Inner self

Energy and Healing

Healing is a natural ability, and we are all naturally healers. We can now measure the body's energy in volts as well as the subtle energy body that is called the aura. Through our conditioning and programming we have allowed our abilities to become blocked, and many have forgotten that we can heal ourselves. According to quantum science, our bodies are "thought energy" living in a sea of energy. We have the ability to become an infinite vortex of the universal life-forces, enabling us to heal ourselves and help others to do the same.

By re-establishing a dynamic "at-one-ment" with our physical, spiritual, intuitive, and creative selves, we become a conduit for the energies of the universe, which would naturally regenerate and rejuvenate us.

WE CAN HEAL OURSELVES!

This connection to the universal life force allows us to direct this energy and transmute ourselves and our environment. By understanding the laws of nature governing the harnessing of this energy, the healer never depletes him/herself of energy and never absorbs the aches and pains of those being helped. Each healing practice becomes a self-energising experience for everyone involved.

To be an effective healer you need to awaken you natural telepathic and empathic abilities. These subtle senses are used to communicate on various subtle levels whilst practising healing. Your subtle senses are like feedback mechanisms that allow you to read the subtle energies beyond the physical reality and allow you to be more in touch with your environment. Many people in the spiritual field think to awaken your subtle senses means you are spiritual—no, you have merely awakened your feedback mechanisms to allow yourself to read your reality on a more subtle level. It is like the dials you have on your car dashboard, which inform you of what is happening with your engine, in the same way your psychic senses are like the lights assisting you in knowing what is happening in your environment more subtly. Through an impeccable attitude, one is able to use one's awakened gifts to make a difference with his or her own inner creative intuitive resources.

SYMPTOMS ARE AN OPPORTUNITY TO LEARN ABOUT OURSELVES...

What is healing? Many believe that it is the removal of disease, energy blocks, and unwanted energies. If you focus on being a healer to remove these aspects, then for you to function as a healer you will need to continue manifesting people who have different types of ailments for you to be in business, therefore perpetuating a reality of disease. In real-

14

ity, you only assist the recipients to suspend their attachment to the ailment to allow the natural life force to flow and create a shift in resonance to be healed. You are creating an opportunity for people to make a different choice and heal themselves. Symptoms are a chance to learn; therefore, removing energy blockages through your yoga practice or through various healing methods without awareness can allow these aliments and blockages to manifest again until you learn from them.

Death is one of the most magnificent initiations we go through and we have been programmed to be afraid of death. Death is something we will all have to come to terms with one day. A lady came to me one day and told me she was dying of cancer and that she had three months to live. I responded, "That's fantastic that you know when you will die; I may have a car accident tonight and not even see tomorrow." I then told her if she was indeed going to die in three months, she has time to prepare herself and say goodbye to everyone. I mentioned that she was privileged because many people don't get the chance to say goodbye and prepare.

Lastly, I offered her the opportunity to live, not being afraid of death, and then perhaps in her last three months (if that was all that she believed she had left) she would be able to truly live life not fearing death. We choose the when, where, how, and why to die, but we can change our minds. Most of us choose to be unaware, and the general program ensures that we waste our life force and only make it to approximately seventy years of age. If people wish to move on to another life (die), as healers we respect this right and it is up to us to help them to move on graciously, perhaps giving them the option that they can die, without creating all the dramas and traumas and to leave elegantly. Like the yogi Paramahansa Yogananda, who on March 7, 1952, went through Mahasamadhi (a yogi's final conscious exit from the body) and died. He chose when, where, how, why, and with whom, and twenty days after his death, his body had not decomposed at all. His body still had the same shine and glow as the moment before he left.

Healing has very little to do with the symptoms. One heals at a consciousness level. As we create our own reality, we end up creating harmony or disharmony within ourselves and this eventually manifests as a symptom, illness, and disease. Symptoms will eventually disappear when one's consciousness changes, i.e., your decisions, attitudes, choices, beliefs, self-image, and perception. This is why it is so important to bring to your awareness the en-

15

…THE BODY SEIZES THIS CHANCE TO TURN ON THE HEALING MECHANISMS. ~RICHARD FAULDS -

LIFE IS NOT, SIMPLY REACHING DEATH IN A SAFE MANNER!

TRANSFORM YOUR RELATIONSHIP WITH YOUR NEGATIVE EGO!

YOGA IS POSSIBLE FOR ANYBODY WHO REALLY WANTS IT. YOGA IS UNIVERSAL.... BUT DON'T APPROACH YOGA WITH A BUSINESS MIND LOOKING FOR WORLDLY GAIN. ~SRI KRISHNA PATTABHI JOIS

ergies you are releasing in the different postures, so that the healing can be on a conscious level, thus allowing you to learn and take your yoga practice to a new level of awareness, knowing yourself and self healing.

Many healers feel special and better than others because of their profession. This includes all spiritual teachers, yoga teachers, all therapists, medical health workers, and alternative therapy healers. This is based upon the negative ego, which creates separation through judgement—feeling "better than" another. yourself and burn out, as the negative ego only wants to set you up to fail and destroy you. So, if we are looking for recognition outside validation (negative ego influence), we limit the amount of energy we can access because the negative ego does not have access to all of your resources.

Living in Touch with Nature

DOES HUMANITY ACTUALLY THINK IT IS EVOLVING THROUGH TECHNOLOGY?

Working with a Tibetan Lama, he has stated that there is a need for people to reconnect with nature. One day as we conversed, he mentioned that humanity thinks they are evolving through technology. Look at what we have done to the planet with our so-called evolved way of thinking. We have polluted the earth, created toxic materials that threaten to poison our world, and created bombs capable of destroying the planet many times over and machines that are replacing people's jobs and creating poverty and desperation while those who create the machinery become exorbitantly wealthy at the expense and expenditure of others. Technology, balanced with Spirituality, is a powerful medium.

ANIMALS RESPOND TO A QUIET MIND...

The intellectual tends to think (which is the real problem) that he or she knows much more than the native cultures. If we place an intellectual who lives in the city out in the bush and leave them there to survive, how long do you feel they will last? Not very long, because they have lost their connection to the elements and nature. Having grown up in the northern part of Australia and Southern Africa, we have had encounters with the shaman and witch doctors who live in harmony with nature. These people know how to live from the land by reading the elements and the land itself. They are very intuitive and sensitive to the environment. In a massive cyclone that struck in Darwin, Australia, in 1974, the ants and birds started leaving the area en mass, up to three days before it happened, and the Aboriginals that were still connected with nature sensed something was coming and they

16 also left the city and went into the bush.

We were told on a recent visit to the USA that fifty years ago 75 percent of people used to live in the rural country area and 25 percent in the cities. Now fifty years later, it has reversed to 25 percent living in the rural country areas and 75 percent in the cities. Most, who have moved to the cities looking for more money, have lost touch with nature and being able to survive off the land and be self-sustainable.

Now they are dependent upon others to grow their food and maintain their lifestyle. With sources of food being contaminated with chemicals and being genetically modified and ending up having a lower nutritional value, this could contribute to many more health problems surfacing. People need access to real organic seeds so they can grow their own food and maintain their health and be self-sustainable. When you learn to put your energy into growing your own food, the plants, being sensitive, respond to what your body needs and the food is much healthier.

Animals can sense the harmony/disharmony within people and an exercise we give students is to sit in the bush and watch the animal's reactions to you. If an animal bolts and runs away, it is because the animal senses the disharmony in you. This is telling you that you need to meditate daily (active meditation is yoga asana; passive meditation is a closed eye experience where you focus on detaching from your mind and body) to quieten and eventually still your mind. Our chaotic thoughts send signals out that frighten nature, and only Masters and people who have done lots spiritual cultivation are able to call birds and wildlife to their hands. Try it out and you will be pleasantly surprised when nature comes calling.

We have experienced wolves, whales, dolphins, lions, humming birds, moose, antelope, zebra, rock rabbits, chipmunks, bears, squirrels and many delightful creatures on our journeys, as they are drawn to our energy. It is available to everyone, it takes work and dedication and a willingness to change your present ideas about nature. Nature holds all the secrets to a beautiful world if only we observe her ways and follow them.

Meditation, Contemplation & Concentration

Meditation is a very important part of yoga and your self-development. What is meditation? Meditation is the act of withdrawing your consciousness of objective reality and exploring your inner reality. It starts with a process of learning to quiet the mind and slowing

LIFE MAY NOT BE THE PARTY WE HOPED FOR, BUT WHILE WE ARE HERE, WE SHOULD DANCE!
- JAYLEE B -

GROWING UP NATURALLLY HAS UNIQUE ADVANTAGES.

down your thought processes until you can stop thinking completely, having no thoughts going through your mind. Once you reach this state you have entered an altered state where you can access cosmic consciousness, sometimes called Samadhi.

When you enter a relaxed state, your conscious mind slows down and you can enter your subconscious and/or your unconscious mind to reprogram how you interact with and access these parts of your mind.

Concentration is a necessary part of meditation because you need to stay focused to develop the power of your will so you cannot be affected and/or distracted by anyone or anything, especially when in a meditative state.

Contemplation is where you are pondering upon something in a neutral state so you can glean more awareness and understanding about a situation or person. Through contemplation you impact upon what you are observing. To stay in a contemplative state you need concentration and willpower. The more you develop your ability for concentration, contemplation, and meditation the easier you will manifest what you want in your yoga practice and within your life.

We heard of a study where it was noticed that when a person is engaged in an act of giving, not only does the person receiving indicate higher levels of serotonin (natural pleasure-enhancing chemicals) but the giver too indicates a spike in serotonin. And to cap it all, a neutral observer, watching the giving, registers a serotonin increase in the brain. So, everyone witnessing the act of giving receives pleasure. In the same way, observing yourself and being aware of your patterns and reactions can benefit you tremendously.

It is important to be unaffected and grounded as you walk through your day. Unaffected does not mean distant or cold, unfeeling or insensitive. It is a state that allows you to feel and release the impact of any situation, without anyone knowing. True meditation is simply the setting aside of your physical body and mind and stepping out. It is your chance to connect with a higher consciousness that is much more than your everyday self and your physical environment and where you can have a glimpse of real freedom.

It takes discipline, focus, concentration, and single-mindedness. The practice of meditation can reveal how distracted you can be and where you are losing energy during the day. Most people can only stay focussed from six to ten seconds and then they are distracted. Einstein could focus single-mindedly for twenty minutes. Contemplation allows the cosmic to communicate with you. It is your chance to be quiet and allow your thoughts to be guided to where you will discover more about yourself.

The Five Minds

There are five different minds: the Superconscious, Unconscious, Subconscious, Conscious, and Animal-level Consciousness.

The animal mind relates to the animal instinct that yogis talk about, being able to withdraw the senses and not allow these drives to control you in life. The body has an instinct to survive, and when you operate from this level you are very animalistic in your behaviour and motives. You respond like the reptiles, being very territorial, controlling, and aggressive. You tend to be focused on the materialistic level, very physically driven, focused upon sex on the physical level mainly, and easily influenced by your body, how it looks, how it feels, its addictions, etc.

When you are practicing yoga or any physical exercise or activity, you need to realize that you need to work with your body and not dominate it. Maintaining correct and safe posture is essential, although you should not force your body into any posture or activity as you can injure yourself and create disharmony within your body. When you end up controlling your body in a dominating way, you create disharmony, and your body will resist and problems can then manifest. This creates tension and eventually something will have to break down. This tension eventually creates energetic imbalances, which manifest as ailments and disease. This includes they way you work with feeding your body. Do you impose a diet or food regime or do you work with your body and understand what it needs and wants? Are you in touch with and can you communicate with your body to know what it wants?

IT TAKES DISCIPLINE, FOCUS, CONCENTRATION AND SINGLE-MINDED NESS.

Quite often we end up forcing food into our bodies at least three times per day, when often we don't really need the food. We have conditioned ourselves to eat too much. The Tibetan Master we work with stated we only need a handful of good food per day to rebuild the wear and tear on the body ever as we absorb prana (life-force) directly from the universe and not from the food we eat. We teach people to bless their food and to put good thoughts into what they eat so it will be better for them.

The conscious mind relates to your everyday thoughts that are being produced by your conditioning and programming from your upbringing. If you have between fifty thousand to eighty thousand thoughts per day, we would like to suggest that 90 percent of them are not yours and they have not originated from your mind but from others.

Your conscious mind is now the part of your mind that has the power to respond and take action. In the past, the power was in your subconscious mind, which determined your responses. Everything is a product of conscious thought and this is referred to in the book called The Secret with the law of attraction. Being conscious means that you can set intention with awareness and be present every moment.

YOU NEED TO WORK WITH YOUR BODY, IT LISTENS AND RESPONDS...

Many high intellectuals are not conscious of what they don't know because they cannot think beyond their dimension of thinking. Einstein stated that "you cannot resolve a situation at the same level of thinking that created it," so you cannot go beyond what you know using the same part of the brain and the same level and way of thinking. You need to be conscious that there is so much more that you do not know then you know and be prepared to explore beyond. To be conscious means to be present in the moment. Realize your conscious mind has access to much less than your subconscious and unconscious minds. So this is how we need to go beyond our limits by going beyond wanting the conscious mind to work out everything.

The subconscious mind filters every experience you have in your present lifetime and changes each lifetime. It contains of all your life's experience, programming, and conditioning. Your subconscious mind is highly emotionally charged, so you need to express and/or neutralise them. Your subconscious mind is the next step in your conscious evolution and you can make turn it into an amazing resource that works for you in everyday life.

Many of your fears come from your parents, your teachers, your religious/spiritual beliefs, and the worldly authorities. All your ugly thoughts and worst fears are there. The subconscious mind does not work within normal time, so anyone can access his or her subconscious mind and tap spiritual awareness in a very short time, whereas some may have been

studying for many years to attain this. The subconscious mind does not operate under the normal rules of life so this can be challenging for some. Within your subconscious mind, you have your true self-image, so do you really want to know yourself as you really are?

Your subconscious mind gathers all your experiences and maintains consistency by filtering all your possible future experiences through your programming, no matter if the programming is negative or positive. Your subconscious mind has access to all information and all the different realms so it is essential for you to work with it. You need to talk to your subconscious mind in symbols and pictures, as those are its language. You also need to communicate with your subconscious mind consciously by talking to it, thanking it for what you have created, and at the same time requesting more. Also use your affirmations in the present tense of "I am" and not "I will."

The unconscious mind relates to the realm of the archetypes. This has been called the collective unconscious where all people's lifetimes exist. All your resources come from the unconscious mind. And so the energies that generate and sustain you are sourced in the unconscious, through the archetypal energies. It is the realm of mythology. Your unconscious mind is the realm of possibility of absolutely everything. Your light and dark side are there.

The super-conscious mind is the mind of God, Goddess, the Source. This level of mind is beyond what we can talk about. It is to be experienced and absorbed. The more you try to talk about this level of mind, the more you limit and restrict it and end up with your personal projection of what you think and feel it is, which separates you from the real thing. It has been linked with the states called Samadhi, Nirvana, and Heaven, among others.

You incarnated into this life with a reasonably clean hard drive, your brain. Then from the moment of birth, you've been programmed and the hard drive has so much software loaded on it now that your computer is running very slow. This download you received created an idea of who you think you are and a new paradigm of how you see yourself and life. You may have heard that you need to lose yourself to find yourself. In order to discover who you are, you need to know what you have become.

You need to lose yourself/your mind (the mind that you have had created for you) to find yourself/true mind. Then you explore the other aspects of your mind, conscious, subconscious, and unconscious. From there you need to lose that mind to connect with "The

Mind," the super-conscious mind, and become one with it.

You need to understand that everything is energy; quantum physicists state this and energy is linked to consciousness. That is why a psychic can hold an object and sense where a person is because the consciousness in the object has a memory and is linked to everything via consciousness. Realising this, you have a body that is mainly filled with water. Dr. Emoto states in his book about water that it is the most sensitive of the elements. If water is programmable with our thoughts, then it stands to reason that our thoughts can program our bodies. What thoughts are you thinking and are they the quality that you want them to be?

Free Will

You have all heard of free will and the fact that everyone has it, but what is it and how do you use it? It obviously has to do with your will and to what extent you will exercise your free will. The two prices you pay for free will are: first, that you have to take responsibility for your reality, and second, that you have to give up your negative ego as your main drive in life.

Our free will assists us to make choices and decisions based upon our own contemplative thought. The negative ego bypasses common sense and produces a static, one-dimensional thought that has been etched into the pathways of the brain. It is the reason for cyclic, reoccurring patterns and experiences. Make a new decision and engage free will.

Going Beyond Past Patterns

If we take a look at our world, many things are breaking down and changing. Change always brings up fears about what will happen because you cannot see the outcome before it happens. The intellectual mind is conditioned to refer to the past and make assessments and evaluate, then plan a course of action. When the intellectual mind doesn't have these reference points it becomes challenged and confused. Exploring the unknown is essential for your development and growth. If you were never to go beyond what you know, you would never grow. Applying this to your yoga, you would never have any progress in a posture because you would stay at the same expression of that particular posture forever. This would become very boring and boredom could eventually destroy you.

When you look at the reason why you respond and function in a habitual way, it is usually because of the intellectual mind. It is easy; it takes no conscious thought on your behalf. You are on autopilot. This is when you are not in touch with life and mistakes and injuries manifest. You also miss out on experiencing more out of life. Habitual patterns relate to addictions. You cannot afford to play around with your development, especially at this time in our evolution, because there is too much at stake and you need to be committed and serious about your development and growth. Be willing to let go of making the past perfect and focus on being present. Often we have an addiction to the past because we are keeping our outlook of people the same to justify our attitude.

Learn to break your habits by tying your shoelaces differently. This was an exercise a master gave me many years ago. I applied it to my shoes and then to the rest of my life. This exercise makes you present in the moment and you learn to do things differently.

A SUCCESSFUL PERSON
IS ONE WHO CAN LAY A
FIRM FOUNDATION
WITH BRICKS THAT
OTHERS THROW AT
THEM.
~ DAVID BRINKLEY -

YOGA, AN ANCIENT BUT PERFECT SCIENCE,
DEALS WITH THE EVOLUTION OF HUMANITY.
THIS EVOLUTION INCLUDES ALL ASPECTS OF ONE'S BEING,
FROM BODILY HEALTH TO SELF-REALIZATION.
YOGA MEANS UNION - THE UNION OF BODY WITH
CONSCIOUSNESS AND CONSCIOUSNESS WITH THE SOUL.
YOGA CULTIVATES THE WAYS OF MAINTAINING
A BALANCED ATTITUDE IN DAY-TO-DAY LIFE AND
ENDOWS SKILL IN THE PERFORMANCE OF ONE'S ACTIONS.
~B.K.S. IYENGAR -

Part Three: The Chakra System

Introduction to the Seven Main Chakras

The word "chakra" comes from Sanskrit and means "wheel" or "vortex of energy." It is an Eastern term given to the vortexes of energy that manifest as spheres of different light vibrations, positioning themselves in the centre of your spinal column. These vortexes of energy are transformers that down step the raw universal life force to specific vibrations that we need to revitalise the different parts of our bodies' systems. They have nothing really to do with the Eastern philosophies except that the term "chakras" was given to them. Through understanding how your chakras work and what they relate to within you, you can access more power, harmony, and completeness.

Contrary to popular belief, there is one set of chakras for all mankind. This set is simply reflected within each human being. Our connection to them depends upon our level of harmony with each one. The clarity and intensity of colour are dependent upon that harmony. At no time can a chakra be closed, only disharmonious, leaving the colour distorted and murky. "Chakras are gateways (vortices of energy) for the etheric energy to enter the physical and for the physical energy to enter the etherium (beyond the physical)," according to The Lazaris Materials' "Healing the Nature of Health." They are the corridors through

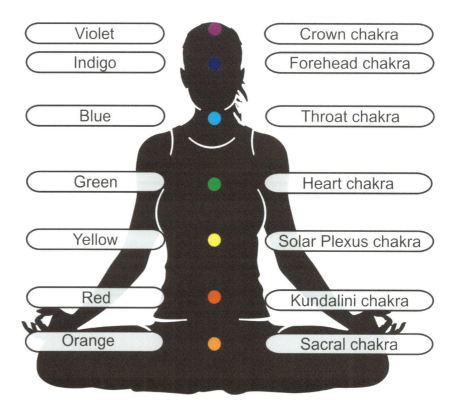

Violet	Crown chakra
Indigo	Forehead chakra
Blue	Throat chakra
Green	Heart chakra
Yellow	Solar Plexus chakra
Red	Kundalini chakra
Orange	Sacral chakra

which all energy, which is in your physical, emotional, mental, and causal systems, pass. The etheric body down steps through the chakras to manifest the aura and the physical body. When doing particular exercises you are activating chakra energies. These exercises can be physical, emotional, and mental through to meditative experiences. Through practicing various yoga asanas, forms of martial arts, and physical exercise you start to release trapped energy and vibrate on different levels of consciousness. This process allows you to receive the energy that is flowing in through the chakras to your physical body more freely and effectively. We can also express and release energy through the chakras, enabling us to function more effectively in the physical realm. Through meditation you are able to balance your chakra energies. Now, let's look at the different chakras giving you an overview of the energies beginning at the base or root chakra, which is called the Kundalini.

Chakra Secret

There has been a lot of confusion with the chakras, which is an interesting manifestation as it relates to security, power, and knowledge. When you look at someone's chakras from the back, the Kundalini is the lowest chakra on the tip of the coccyx and the Sacral chakra is situated in the lower back (see insert). From the front the sacral chakra, being an orange glow, is at the groin, and there is the reflection of the Kundalini above the Sacral chakra just below the navel. It is sometimes referred to as the Midpoint, Hara, and some even call it the spleen chakra or lower abdomen chakra. The spleen is just below your left breast and it has its own chakra and glow there.

Many have written on the chakras and haven't really known or could not really see the chakras. Few know that the Kundalini projects into the front of the body just below the navel and above the genitals and is the size approximately of an apple or a clenched fist. The colour of this sphere is ruby red. To ground yourself, simply bring your awareness to the area below your navel. It is a practice used by martial artists.

The Sacral projects downwards into the genitals and you will discover a tiny glow where the ovaries are too. It is little wonder that during menstruation most women suffer with lower back issues. If you look at society as a whole, where do you find the greatest amount of distortion? Sex and power! These two chakras have revealed an age-old secret and understanding into the distortion.

27

YOGA TEACHES US TO CURE WHAT NEED NOT BE ENDURED AND ENDURE WHAT CANNOT BE CURED.
~B.K.S. IYENGAR -

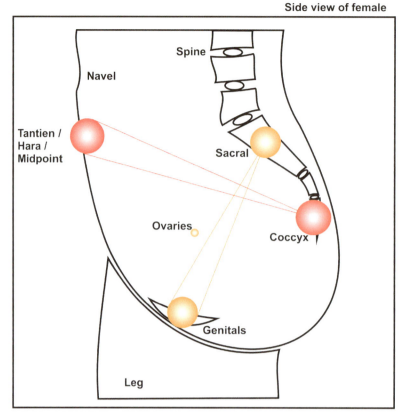

Side view of female

Spine

Navel

Tantien /
Hara /
Midpoint

Sacral

Ovaries

Coccyx

Genitals

Leg

Perhaps there is more than meets the eye? Consider your own life and where you have had the most adversity. Power and sex have brought nations to their knees; presidents have fallen and great leaders have been dethroned because power has been used to gain sex and sex used to gain power.

Corresponding Chakras in Limbs and Torso

Chakras have correspondences in the limbs and imbalances in the chakras can play out in the associating areas in the limbs. Although the mathematics behind the chakras is vast, we will only look at three layers of the chakras in this book. Namely, the main chakra energies, the secondary correspondences in the limbs, and tertiary correspondences in the entire body. It is important to remember that each chakra impacts the other six. Combine the Kundalini with the Sacral chakra and you can see immediately the cross pollination of power through sexuality. Combine the Solar Plexus with the Kundalini and you get emotional power. With this in mind, it is not hard to see how we observed and experienced the multi-dimensional quality of the chakra system. Using only these three layers, there are 144 different reflections taking place.

The following is a look at secondary connections:

The Main Kundalini chakra is reflected in the hands and feet. Problems with these areas would result from imbalances in this chakra.

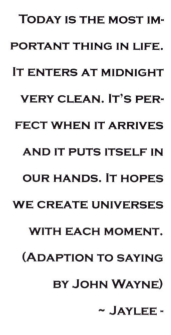

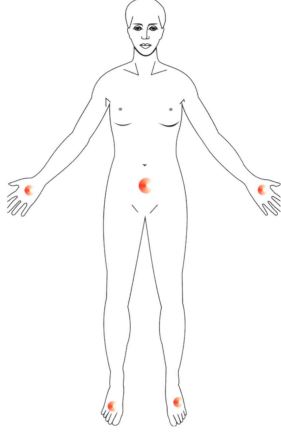

The main Sacral chakra is reflected in the wrists and ankles. Problems with these areas would result from imbalances in this chakra.

IF I'M LOSING BALANCE
IN A POSE,
I STRETCH HIGHER AND
GOD REACHES DOWN
TO STEADY ME.
 IT WORKS EVERY TIME,
AND NOT JUST IN YOGA.
~TERRI GUILLEMETS -

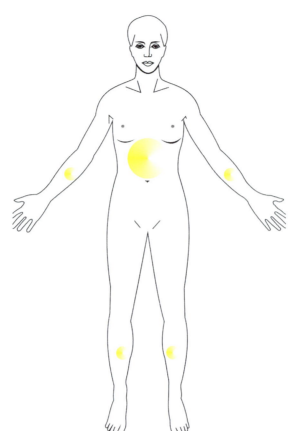

The main Solar Plexus chakra is reflected in the forearms and calves. Problems with these areas would result from imbalances in this chakra.

The main Heart chakra is reflected in the elbows and knees. Problems with these areas would result from imbalances in this chakra.

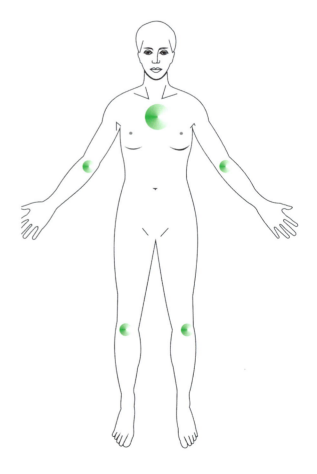

YOU HAVE FOLLOWED THE PATH OF SOMEONE ELSE, LEARN NOW TO CREATE YOUR OWN
- PAUL G BALCH

The main Throat chakra is reflected in the shoulders and hips. Problems with these areas would result from imbalances in this chakra.

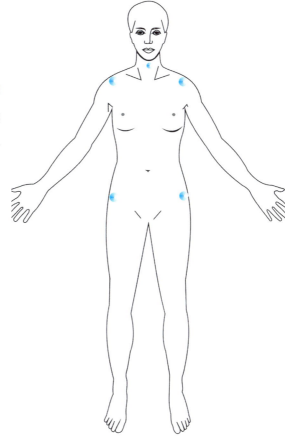

The Main Forehead and Crown chakra have no other corresponding reflections within the human body.

"WE ARE PART OF THE WHOLE WHICH WE CALL THE UNIVERSE, BUT IT IS AN OPTICAL DELUSION OF OUR MIND THAT WE THINK WE ARE SEPARATE. THIS SEPARATENESS IS LIKE A PRISON FOR US. OUR JOB IS TO WIDEN THE CIRCLE OF COMPASSION SO WE FEEL CONNECTED TO ALL PEOPLE AND ALL SITUATIONS."
~ ALBERT EINSTEIN -

The following is a look at tertiary connections:

(Excerpts from - Healing the Nature of Health recording: www.lazaris.com)

The FEET can reflect Kundalini Energy

The SHINS and CALVES can reflect Sacral Energy

The THIGHS and HAMSTRINGS can reflect Solar Plexus Energy

The PELVIS can reflect Heart Energy

The TORSO can reflect Throat Energy

The SIXTH and SEVENTH Energy Centres are NOT reflected in the physical body at all.

Explanation on the Three Chakra Layers

Given the three layers previously shown—the primary chakras, secondary correspondences in the limbs, and tertiary correspondences in the whole body, it is easy to see that there are many overlapping energies to take into consideration.

The pelvic area, for example, has:

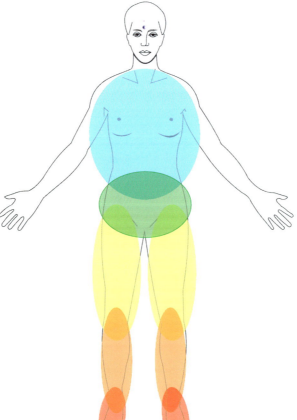

Primary Chakras: Kundalini and Sacral (power and creativity)

Secondary Correspondences: Throat chakra (hips)

Tertiary Correspondences: Heart chakra (green area) - (see insert)

In the pelvic area alone, four chakra energies are interlinked. This is why it is seen as the Seat of the Self or where we express or manifest our self-image, self-worth, self-esteem, and self-importance. It is also important to note that the main pivot point in yoga is the pelvic region. It connects our legs with the rest of our body!

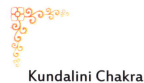

Kundalini Chakra

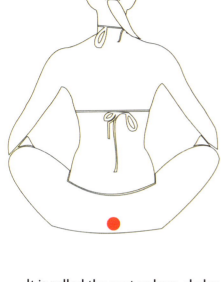

Known as: Muladhara , root, kundalini, base centre

Where: End of coccyx, perineum, hands, feet, below navel

Affects: obesity, haemorrhoids, constipation, sciatica

Main energy: security, grounding, safety

It is called the root or base chakra and is positioned on the tip of the coccyx. If you remember in the Bible when Eve ate of the fruit of the tree of knowledge (good and evil), it was symbolizing that humanity was accessing their Kundalini energy. The Kundalini energy in general relates to security, safety, and balance. Issues with your feet and hands relate to insecurities and imbalances in the Kundalini energy. It manifests in the following ways: You're afraid you are will not be able to stand your ground in a situation, you are afraid you are going to fall on your butt, you don't feel firmly grounded in a situation, you are afraid you will not be able to hold on to what to have, or something is beyond your grasp. You ask yourself, Do we have enough money, health, will the relationship last, will my career last?

These are all issues relating to security and your language builds on your energy. For example, Athlete's foot, haemorrhoids, and poison oak on your hands could relate to issues of security and Kundalini imbalances. It has a sense of earnestness; determination, or focusing and self-reliance. After you have willed something, you follow it through. It is the seat of your security.

One of the imbalances relates to chauvinism, seeing men as idiots or judging and having a hatred for women. It is also your power, the source of your life force within the physical world, and it also relates to wisdom and knowledge (as the coiled serpent in various symbols). It also relates to the fruit in the tree of knowledge, where humanity accepted their power, choice, and free will to experience duality by accepting the fruit of the tree of life, of good and evil. The fruit has been seen as a red apple, which represents the Kundalini energy and power. When you focus in your head (intellect), you're not in touch with your power and with what's going on; you don't have much power to resist. When you're concentrating on that midpoint 50 millimeters below your navel, you're grounded and in touch with your power.

The seven levels of the Kundalini Energy:

First level relates to: Are you secure enough to feel secure?

Second level relates to: Are you secure enough to be creative, sexual, and have fun?

Third level relates to: Are you secure to be honest and emotionally vulnerable?

Fourth level relates to: Are you secure enough to love and be intimate?

Fifth level relates to: Are you secure enough to communicate and express yourself?

Sixth level relates to: Are you secure enough to have a vision and be intuitive?

Seventh level relates to: Are you secure enough to access your unlimited potential in the ethereal world (beyond the physical)?

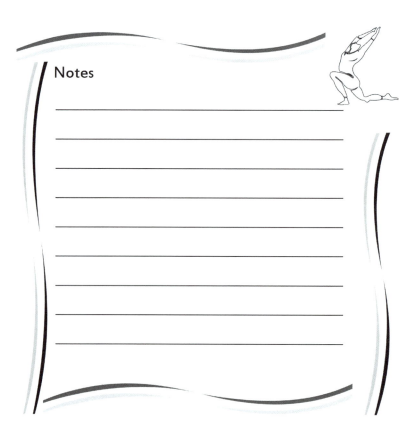

Notes

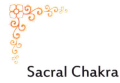

Sacral Chakra

Known as: Svadhisthara, sacral centre

Where: between legs, sacrum,
   reproductive system, wrists, ankles

Affects: desire, pleasure, creativity,
   reproductive system, impotence,
   frigidity

Main energy: pleasure, sexuality, creativity

It is the sacral energy that manifests in the sacrum, lower back, and the genital area of the groin. In women it includes the ovaries and in men the testes. Injuries and weakness with your ankles and wrists relate to a difficulty with pleasure. This also relates to sexual pleasure and when manifesting a sexual disease, this often relates to sexual guilt.

This also encompasses problems with the prostate gland in men.

The second chakra relates to creativity, pleasure, and sexuality. Sex is not the only form of pleasure we can experience. Everything that has to do with pleasure in your life relates to the second chakra. Pleasure in creating, having fun, being alive, and doing what makes us happy is all related to pleasure. The ankles relate to sexual stability and feeling sexually loved. Over the years we have seen countless manifestations of difficulties with pleasure and the results thereof.

The knowledge in this material is not to challenge you but to awaken your awareness to think deeper and realise that physical ailments manifest for reasons beyond the normal diagnosis. If you have an ailment or have had an injury, just contemplate where you could have more pleasure and get this knowledge to work for you instead of reacting to it. For example, runners develop shin splints, often related to a difficulty in having pleasure as they issues around receiving pleasure.

Movies, food, reading, sex, crafts, fun, and music all relate to this chakra. Usually you aren't letting it in, you don't like it, you're afraid of it, you think you don't deserve it, or you're afraid you are going to get punished for it. many people work until they drop, but seldom sit back and enjoy the fruits of their labour.

The seven levels of the Sacral energy:

First level relates to: Do you feel joy in your security?

Second level relates to: Do you feel joy in sexuality and fun?

Third level relates to: Do you feel joy in being honest and emotionally vulnerable?

Fourth level relates to: Do you feel joy in love and intimacy?

Fifth level relates to: Do you feel joy in communicating and expressing?

Sixth level relates to: Do you feel joy in your intuition and internal wisdom?

Seventh level relates to: Do you feel joy in connecting with your unlimited potential in the ethereal world (beyond the physical)?

Notes

_____

_____

_____

_____

_____

_____

_____

_____

_____

Solar Plexus Chakra

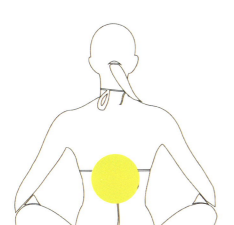

Known as: Manipura, solar plexus centre

Where: Solar plexus, digestive system,
forearms, calves

Affects: pancreas, stomach, liver, gall
bladder & nervous system

Main energy: feeling feelings, willpower,
vulnerability, honesty

 This is dealing with accumulating and transforming the emotions; it is the emotional centre. Issues with your calves, shins, and forearms relate to the issues of emotional control. Shins relate to frustration and calves relate to emotional instability.

The third chakra has to do with control issues. It begins with manipulative control and rises to creative control or creative generation. Manipulative control can wound others and although you get what you want, you seldom gain a true sense of self. Creative control is far grander and allows you to use your emotions to support your intentions. Therefore it is the chakra of honesty and vulnerability. If you are honest with yourself and express your emotions without judgment, you gradually allow yourself to show vulnerability. Vulnerability is a strength in the right circumstance and with the right person.

This chakra has to do with the processing of and dealing with emotions. When we can't handle processing and letting go of our emotions we end up stuffing them within our bodies. It relates to all the emotions, the so=called positive and negative ones that you refuse to become vulnerable to. The full range of emotions is connected to this chakra. What is important here is that no emotions are actually negative, although it is referred to many books. Emotions are energy in motion. A negative emotion is simply one that has not been expressed. You have judged it and it has become trapped in your body. A trapped emotion is like stagnant water; it becomes putrefied and acidic and can cause many physical ail-

37

ments. Expressing anger and fear can serve as the fuel for cleaning the house, gardening, and plunging through a project that you have left for months.

You should continuously expand your range of feeling emotions, from the most expansive to the most contracting, from the most beautiful to the ugliest. The key here is to release all emotions in an elegant and constructive way. Do yoga, scream in a pillow, hug a person, write about what you feel, run a mile, or sing. Just express and move! Screaming at a partner or physically abusing someone is not elegant and can result in trouble. It is all about emotional management.

I heard a Tao master state, that when a Tao master dies their body never go into rigor mortis. Why? Because they spend their lives expressing, purging, cleansing, and detoxing all impure emotions/thoughts and attachments, and this allows nothing to be left trapped in their bodies.

The seven levels of the Solar Plexus:

First level relates to: What emotions are triggered regarding your security?

Second level relates to: What emotions are triggered regarding your creativity and pleasure?

Third level relates to: What emotions are triggered regarding expanding the range of your feelings?

Fourth level relates to: What emotions are triggered regarding feeling love and intimacy?

Fifth level relates to: What emotions are triggered regarding your communication and expression?

Sixth level relates to: What emotions are triggered through your intuition and internal wisdom?

Seventh level relates to: What emotions are triggered through connecting with your unlimited potential in the ethereal world (beyond the physical)?

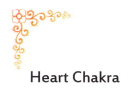

Heart Chakra

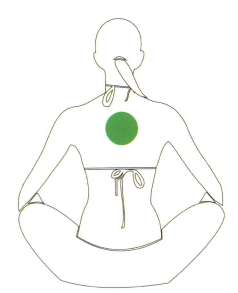

Known as: Anahata, heart centre

Where: Centre of chest, thymus, elbows, knees

Affects: Blood pressure, heart and lungs, touch and equilibrium, thymus

Main energy: intimacy (into-me-see), love

This chakra is positioned in the centre of your chest and relates to your heart. Pelvic area imbalances exist because people get mixed up with love being sex. Women often go from one partner to another wanting love and offering sex in exchange. They are not the same energy.

The heart chakra dynamically puts into action that part of you that takes ideas, creates them, and applies them. It allows you to take ideas and act upon them. The stagnation that comes from unrealised dreams and fantasies has to do with an energy where you hope that someday you are going to be something but that day never comes because you never take any action.

This heart chakra, of course, is love. Love from the simplest survival, love of the infant for mother's milk, to cosmic love that moves beyond that of even humanity, to a love of all there is. If you have problems with your elbows, knees, or your pelvic girdle you have difficulties with love. Giving and receiving love relates to your elbows and ailments attached to them. Give yourself-love first and then give to others. You cannot give what you don't have, and often people look for love outside themselves, which creates co-dependencies with others. Self-love must precede giving love.

The knees identify issues with relationships, especially regarding anger and resentment

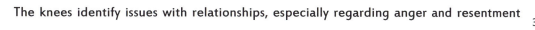

from the past. The left relates to relationships with women and the right with men. Look at mother and father figures or partners in your path to heal.

Love is the most powerful force and is talked about in every corner of life. Most are afraid of and resist love, thinking they don't deserve to be loved. Many are unwilling to give it or receive it and believe love means pain and hurt. Heart and lung issues can relate to the fear or inability to express love and the trapped emotion finds itself impacting the very organ it was meant to move through—the heart. The lungs can relate to a feeling of not being valuable in your world and having a license to be yourself and live freely. This is strongly connected to self-love.

It is the seat of the soul and the point through which unconditional love flows. It is our link with the Cosmic or Soul connection. Through being motivated out of love, it is the chakra where you can connect with the whole. Love is the force that is creating unity and oneness. If you connect with this chakra, you connect with everything and you realise we are everything. Your soul records every first experience you ever had. It does not record repeats or addictions or habits or patterns. These remain in Cosmic Memory for eternity!

The seven levels of the Heart:

First level relates to: Do you feel love for security?

Second level relates to: Do you love your creativity and pleasure?

Third level relates to: Do you feel love for emotions?

Fourth level relates to: Do you love to love and be loved?

Fifth level relates to: Do you love to express and communicate?

Sixth level relates to: Do you love your intuition and internal wisdom?

Seventh level relates to: Do you love through your unlimited potential in the ethereal world
        (beyond the physical)?

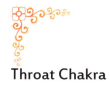

Throat Chakra

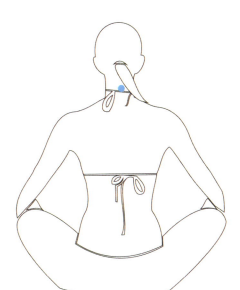

Known as: Visudhha, throat centre

Where: Throat, thyroid, shoulders, hips

Affects: Expression, communication, perception, precognition, telepathic communication, metabolism

Main energy: Expression and communication

This chakra relates to expression and communication, and it is positioned in the centre of your throat over your thyroid gland. Issues with your fifth chakra can manifest as sore throat, issues with your thyroid gland and speaking, and relate to difficulties in communicating and expressing on many levels in life. This chakra expresses everything that is connected to all your energies in the physical and beyond. It is the highest of the physical chakras.

As it is the gateway to expression and related to all the chakras below and above, it is vital in the process of interaction and expression. The corresponding places in the shoulders and hips mean this chakra connects physically with each chakra below it: how we express security (Kundalini), how we express sexuality (Sacral), how we express emotions (Solar Plexus), etc. When we cannot feel our emotions and we cannot express them, we find ourselves weighed down with stagnant energies.

The seven levels of the Throat:

First level relates to: How do you express your security?

Second level relates to: How do you express your fun, pleasure, and sexuality?

Third level relates to: How do you express your emotions?

Fourth level relates to: How do you express your love and intimacy?

NEVER LOOK BACK
UNLESS YOU'RE PLAN-
NING TO GO THAT WAY.

- UNKNOWN -

Fifth level relates to: How do you express yourself?

Sixth level relates to: How do you express your intuition and internal wisdom?

Seventh level relates to: How do you express your unlimited potential in the ethereal world (beyond the physical)?

Notes

_____

_____

_____

_____

_____

_____

_____

_____

_____

_____

Forehead Chakra

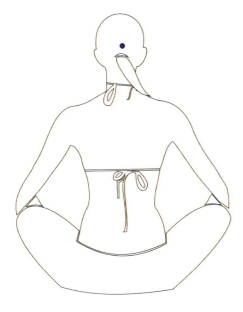

Known as: Ajna, third Eye, brow, forehead centre

Where: Forehead, pituitary gland

Affects: Intuition, internal dialogue, free will, choice, dreams

Main energy: Awareness, intuition

This chakra relates to psychic awareness and intuition. It is positioned inside your forehead and is approximately 2.5 centimeters inside your skull. It relates to your internal vision, intuition and psychic awareness, the awakenings, epiphanies, and wisdom. This is the bridge! It relates to that part of you that can see beyond the current picture to the bigger picture, without losing sight of the present. This is where you receive intuition from the heavens and bring it down to earth—as above, so below.

The sixth chakra is your intuitive centre, your psychic awareness and psychic centre. The sixth chakra is the doorway to the higher planes. It relates to the pituitary gland. This chakra also relates to your telepathic abilities of thought transference and thought reception. It is possible to send and receive thoughts from anywhere in the universe. Most people have sung a tune in their heads and when they have begun to sing out loud, someone else has claimed to be singing the same song. This energy centre relates to your ability to focus and maintain intention. A strong will and laser-sharp focus are some of the qualities of working with this chakra. It is not until you get to the door of the seventh chakra that you touch your spirituality by reaching the true third eye, which has been called the celestial eye, which is all seeing beyond physical sight and beyond.

 Perhaps headaches and migraines can be caused by not connecting with your inner voice. Strokes manifest because most people think and plan without actually listening to their inner voice. Intense thought can bring much stress. Think about this: What we want is up to us, how we get there is not. So, put that clutch in and allow the heavens to show you the way. Thinking about how may produce some sort of solution, but it may very well not be the most elegant and joyful one. The sixth chakra located in the brow is the centre of psychic awareness, intuition, and wisdom. It scans your futures for anything that can assist in developing your intuition and higher faculties.

The seven levels of the Forehead:

First level relates to: Do your intuitions bring you security?

Second level relates to: do your intuitions bring you pleasure?

Third level relates to: Do your intuitions allow you to expand your ability to feel?

Fourth level relates to: Do your intuitions allow you to expand your ability to love and be intimate?

Fifth level relates to: Do your intuitions allow you to expand your ability to communicate and express?

Sixth level relates to: Do your intuitions allow you to expand your psychic abilities?

Seventh level relates to: Do your intuitions allow you to tap your unlimited potentials?

Notes

_____

_____

_____

_____

_____

_____

_____

_____

_____

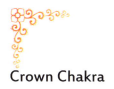

Crown Chakra

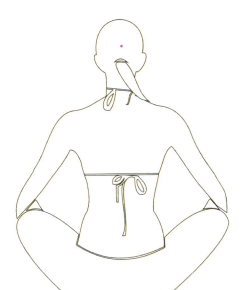

Known as: Sahasrara, celestial eye, crown centre

Where: Pineal gland, middle of brains between hemispheres

Affects: Unlimited potential, harmony and balance

Main energy: Gateway to enlightenment, spiritual door to beyond

This chakra relates to your unlimited potential. It is positioned inside your skull in the middle of your brains approximately 5 centimetres down from the top of your skull, and it is the size of a pea. This chakra relates to a doorway to the spiritual world and accessing your unlimited potential and has also been called the celestial eye. It connects with your pineal gland.

This is where you reach for "home" or the heavens and go beyond the duality of your reality. The seventh chakra, which is located in the centre of the brain, and what you see with it, is what you manifest in this reality.

When you project a vision from your inner eye, it is released to the causal realms and then it returns with the manifestation of what you have projected, good or bad. It is from this chakra that you have out-of-body soul experiences. It is also the centre through which you depart when you die.

The pineal gland of the seventh is linked to the optic nerve indirectly. There are levels to each chakra and there are seven levels to each of them. You won't tap into this level while you are in the physical body.

The seven levels of the Pineal:

First level relates to: Does your unlimited potential allow you security?

Second level relates to: Does your unlimited potential allow you creativity ?

Third level relates to: Does your unlimited potential allow you to expand your range of feeling emotions?

Fourth level relates to: Does your unlimited potential allow you love and intimacy?

Fifth level relates to: Does your unlimited potential allow you expression and communication?

Sixth level relates to: Does your unlimited potential allow you intuition?

Seventh level relates to: Does your unlimited potential allow you to go beyond the physical realms?

The Emotional Organs

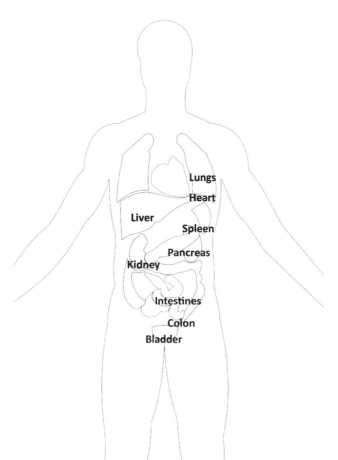

Lungs
Heart
Liver
Spleen
Pancreas
Kidney
Intestines
Colon
Bladder

The LUNGS relate to energy. If you have fear, you can manifest asthma and bronchial conditions. Look at bronchitis.

The HEART is where you begin to feel, and allow all emotions to move through you without judgement. Look at heart attacks and related issues.

The LIVER is where you process your emotions, feel them and let them go. If you don't let go, you can end up with liver problems. Look at alcohol abuse.

The SPLEEN is where we store our resentments and bitterness and relates to our aspirations.

We store anxiety in our STOMACHS. Look at ulcers.

The KIDNEYS relate to the fear of change and rocking the boat. We do not want to appear different or have our own opinions. Look at infections and Adrenal fatigue.

The PANCREAS is where we store those feelings. Look at when you are being too sweet or nice and you are martyring yourself. Be mindful not to give until it hurts. Look at diabetes.

The INTESTINE has to do with gaining nutrition thus gaining value and letting yourself really own something.

The COLON has to do with security; both diarrhoea and constipation have to do with insecurity. Either holding on to past issues or forcefully trying to let go of the past.

The BLADDER relates to disappointment and expectations. Look at infections.

"AT THE HEART OF EACH OF US, WHATEVER OUR IMPERFECTIONS, THERE EXISTS A SILENT PULSE OF PERFECT RHYTHM, A COMPLEX OF WAVE FORMS AND RESONANCES WHICH IS ABSOLUTELY INDIVIDUAL AND UNIQUE, AND YET WHICH CONNECTS US TO EVERYTHING IN THE UNIVERSE."
~ GEORGE LEONARD -

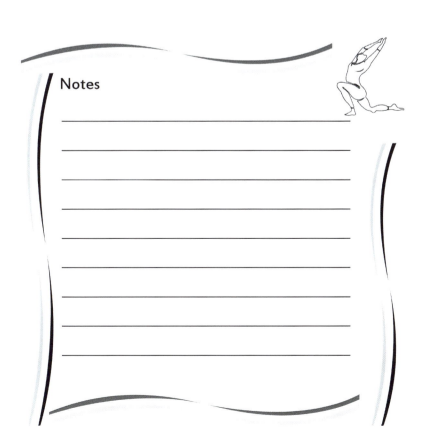

Notes

_____

_____

_____

_____

_____

_____

_____

_____

_____

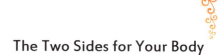

"IF WE HAVE NO PEACE
IT IS BECAUSE WE HAVE
FORGOTTEN THAT
WE BELONG TO EACH
OTHER."
~ MOTHER TERESA -

Your RIGHT side:

Masculinity

Conscious Mind

Doing

Giving

Intending

Form

Actual

Thinking

Father

Males

Check your balance—which side is weaker? Which side is easier? Which is less flexible and uncoordinated? Are you a thinking or feeling person? The side that seems weaker or less balanced is the side you need to integrate. As females, you may find that your right side is weaker or rigid. As males, you may find your left side is more challenging in general.

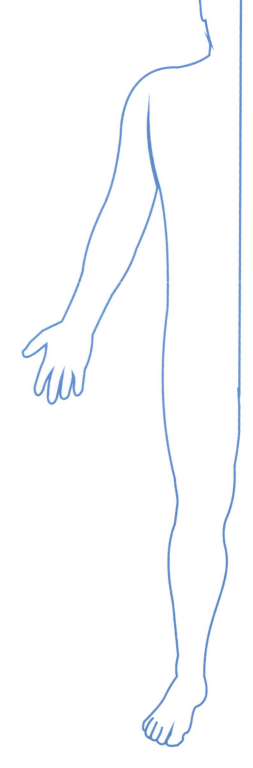

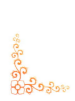

(frontal view)

Your LEFT side:

Femininity

Sub-Conscious Mind

Being

Receiving

Allowing

Chaos

Potential

Feeling

Mother

Females

It is a natural phenomena in yoga that if you have deeply buried issues and your left side lacks balance or you have discomfort, for that to go and to reappear on your right-hand side in the same place. Once an issue is released out of the subconscious mind, it often moves to your conscious mind first, before it is released completely. Never give up!

"AT THE ROOT OF OUR NEED TO CONTROL WE FIND FEAR. IT MAY BE FEAR OF THE UNKNOWN. FEAR OF NOT COPING. FEAR OF LOSS. OR POSSIBLY EVEN FEAR OF LOOK-ING STUPID. AND AS OUR EFFORTS TO CON-TROL OTHER PEOPLE AND EVENTS INVARI-ABLY FAIL, OUR FEAR INCREASES. TRUST, ON THE OTHER HAND, IS A QUALITY OF THE SOUL. WHILE CON-TROL IS A TOOL OF THE MIND, TRUST AND FAITH ARE ASPECTS OF THE HEART. WHEN WE TRUST IN LIFE ENOUGH TO GIVE UP OUR NEED FOR CONTROL, WE CAN RELAX AND OPEN TO THE FLOW OF ENERGY IN OUR LIVES. THIS BRINGS PEACE OF MIND."
~ THE DAILY GURU -

The Celestial Symphony

Once upon a musical, as God wrote my song

God was very excited, the notes played along

The bass, the symbol, the harp stood tall

Such harmony flowed in the celestial hall

I stood there watching the music dance

Hoping, wishing for my lifetime's chance

On and on and into the eternal forever

I stood on the side thinking now or never

I made a move and God stilled my soul

"Be patient child, I`ve planned your role"

The orchestra thundered and the worlds began

From creation to creation the songs sang

At first and last, the universe was placed

A cosmic coliseum, the symphony embraced

A hand swept down and love filled my heart

I had seen the lyrics of God, from the start

"Now is your chance, little angel of mine"

I rose, I sang to the pathway of the divine

I joined the notes from the rock of all ages

From galaxies and worlds unfurled the stages

Of a celestial plan, where God knew the song

Where every note counted, as God sang along

Now every single soul is a part, is a key

Of the Creator's incredible Celestial Symphony

-Jaylee Balch-

PART FOUR: THE ENERGETICS OF POSTURES

Fear is an emotion that we all have in common, and for many it becomes a prison. Fear is an energy that creates separation, often leaving us feeling alone and lonely. Fear is anything that creates a threat physically, emotionally, mentally, or spiritually. It is a part of our mind that seeks to alienate us from the oneness with everything. For many, it is automatic, uncontrollable, paralysing, and becomes the normal response to avoid any environment that hints of its potential.

Within each one of us is the potential to release our fears; however, the easier path most often taken is the lack of willingness to ask the right questions, and then to take the steps to change the condition and gain the understanding needed.

Fear does have a beneficial side, as it can be a very powerful motivator that keeps us focused on what we need to be doing, rather than surrendering and becoming overwhelmed. Fear is a survival instinct and an automatic response and allows us to go into flight or fight mode.

When it becomes seductive and dangerous is when it is blown out of proportion and forms a neurotic perception regarding parts of our reality. For example, if I have fear of spiders, that's fair enough, especially if I have had a bad experience where one bit me or jumped on my face; however, if I have no such memories and I have a terror—enough to make me lose my mind temporarily—I have lost the ability to keep the fear in its right perspective. It has become bigger than an initial fear, and therefore the fear has imprisoned me.

In the limbic system in the brain, where the amygdala sits, being a small gland behind the frontal lobe, this gland triggers the flight or fight response to maintain survival. Fear can be a wake-up call to maintain staying focused, to face and respond to a situation, and to respond to the need for change in your life. Often the fear of the unknown traps you in maintaining the status quo and settling for a mediocre life. The altered ego will often use fear to sabotage you and stop you in your tracks.

Fear can be a valuable feedback mechanism, warning you to know what you are doing and stay focused. Many people fear being exposed because many don't really know who they really are, so being exposed would reveal the lie that you thought you knew who you were, but that was not real. If you leave fear unchecked, it will continue to grow until it paralyses you. Then you end up constantly expecting things to go wrong because it has become part of your identity.

You can learn to face your fears and develop yourself; you reach a place where you can transcend all fear and live a life in a state having a pure heart and mind. This is the state that all spiritual masters live in, a state where they are incapable of feeling fear because they have transcended merely surviving and are spiritually living life to the fullest.

Fear can be likened to a filter or lens, through which we view certain parts of our reality. Most of our reality is calm, normal, and manageable; however, certain parts are viewed through this lens and it distorts and magnifies them, leaving us weak, incapacitated, and powerless. The first step to reclaiming what fear has taken from you is to put the fear in the right perspective—you may need the help of an objective, external person for this—and then to maintain seeing the fear as it arises through the correct lens. So a magnified fear becomes a normal fear. Then, the hard work begins—finding a state of mind where you are fearless in the situation and powerful.

What is interesting is that in our experience there are three main fears that are most likely to have come from the movement experienced through birth: fear of the dark, heights, and confined spaces. They can all be related to the experience of a spirit moving down the birth canal, the spirit falling into a body and being in the tight space.

Practical exercises addressing FEAR:

Exercise: Become aware of your fears—name three on paper.

Exercise: Begin to notice where your fears are controlling your life and to what degree you change, and plan and make decisions around those fears. (For instance—a spider fear would have the person avoiding dark places, checking cupboards, and always wearing shoes.)

Exercise: Trace back where this fear may have been triggered in your life.

> THE GIVER OF A GIFT, THE RECEIVER OF A GIFT AND THE OBSERVER OF THE ACT OF GIVING THE GIFT - ALL RECEIVE THE SAME BENEFIT... CALLED SEROTONIN.
> —*STUDIES IN QUANTUM MECHANICS*

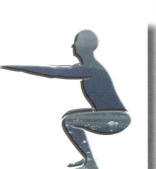

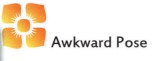

Awkward Pose

Utkatasana

Where do you feel it? Thighs, shoulders, hips, feet, toes, knees?

In the first part of Awkward Pose (see insert), you are working the IT Band (Ilio Tibial Band is a tough group of fibres that run along the outside of the thigh) and working the thigh helps to release anger towards yourself and towards others. Ultimately, all anger is self-anger.

ALLOW NOTHING TO STEAL YOUR PEACE...

As an example: My wife gets angry and lashes out at me. I allow that to affect me. Then I in turn react back. I have absorbed her anger, and not only have I absorbed her anger, but I am angry with myself for allowing that to happen. I have let myself down. I don't want to take responsibility and ownership that I have chosen and allowed it to happen. I then project it back to her, thinking it is her fault. If you project the anger back at the other person by abusing them, you create a perpetuating cycle and it continues. With the energies nowadays, people can project so quickly without first stopping to think. I got affected, I should take responsibility. It has nothing to do with her; I have been shown where I have a weakness. Now I can work on it to heal.

You spend your whole life defending yourself. You desperately try to avoid confrontation. Instead, have the attitude of: "Wow! It has triggered something within me and now I can look at where I can strengthen and be unaffected." All anger comes back to you. People want to feed on energy. They create a situation so that you react and then they get their fix. Allow nothing to steal your peace!

ALL ANGER IS SELF ANGER...

A relationship sits in the space between two people. You cannot take anything from the other person. You can only offer the qualities you want, into the space between yourself and your partner. Your partner then chooses what he or she wants to receive. If you do the same, the space between you becomes the relationship. Love does not bind, it sets free. This counts for all relationships, even platonic ones.

In the second part of Awkward Pose (see insert), you come up on your toes and work deeply into your ankles. When you work the toes, you activate the creative life force, sexual, creative, and fun centre. Number one mandate in spirituality: Have fun.

54

You are working into the ankles, which relates to sexual security and sexual anger in this

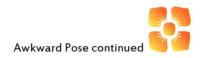
posture. Why would you have sexual anger?

Do you know how you work? Do you know what does it for you, have you explored what you like, and have you expressed that to your partner and what your needs and wants are in the sexual arena? If you haven't, you may be angry with your partner that they don't know how you work and what you want. Hopefully, in the darkness, they fumble and can work out how it all works (chuckle). Sometimes, that is also too easy, so let's have a bottle of wine and a joint and then let's try to make it happen. It is easy to unite the two bodies, but the ultimate connection is the uniting of the physical, emotional, mental, and spiritual bodies. We know how to unite the genitals and create a baby. It's too easy—let's create on the other levels, have a true connection, something of substance and depth. You can have sexual anger because your needs are not being met, but there is a responsibility for you to communicate your needs.

In the third part of Awkward Pose (see insert), when you bring your knees together and you go down into the posture, you are activating the knees, hips, and pelvic area, but this time you are focussing a lot more on the inner thighs, and what you are releasing there is guilt and sexual guilt. All aspects of spirituality have a golden thread of truth, but they don't cultivate self-awareness, and guilt is often a result of taking on the more common spiritual paradigm.

Guilt is a man-made emotion and it is not real. It has no constructive side to it and is only a destructive emotion. Guilt is a lid that you place on your anger. You are made to feel guilty for being angry and it stops you from expressing anger. Many people have layers and layers of anger that they have suppressed because they feel guilty for feeling angry. This often leads to depression. If you get caught in depression you can end up spiralling down and down. If you feel angry, express it constructively!

Often we are told what to do as a child and our own dreams are forfeited. Our parents' dreams for us are acknowledged and our own discarded. We feel angry, but we are not allowed to feel angry towards our parents so we automatically feel guilty about our anger and suppress it. We honour our parents' dreams for us at our own expense. This can lead to depression later in life.

TRUE CHARACTER IS REVEALED WHEN SOMEONE IS ANGRY, NOT WHEN THEY ARE HAPPY
- JAYLEE B -

GUILT IS A MAN - MADE EMOTION...

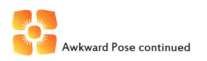

(Insert)

A - Release anger
B - Release sexual anger
C - Release Guilt

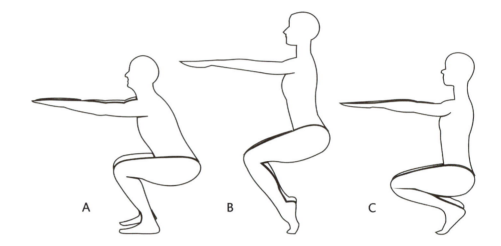

A   B   C

HEALING CONSIDERATIONS:

RECOGNISE AND DEAL WITH ANGER

RELEASE RAGE AND DEEP, HEAVY EMOTIONS

ALLOW YOURSELF TO FEEL ANGRY AND LET GO

RECOGNISE THE HURT CHILD WITHIN AND WORK WITH IT

BALANCE YOUR HYPER SENSITIVITY

RELEASE SEXUAL ANGER FROM NOT HAVING YOUR NEEDS MET

RELEASE GUILT—AN ENERGY THAT CREATES DISHARMONY BETWEEN

YOUR INTERNAL WORLD AND EXTERNAL WORLD.

FOCUS ON CREATING BEAUTIFUL SYNERGIES

EXPRESS YOURSELF AND FEEL COMFORTABLE WITH WHO YOU ARE

Balancing Stick Pose

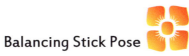
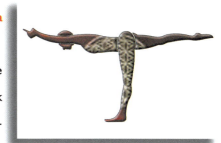

I am sure you are aware that your heart starts to go crazy—it is a very intense heart posture. You are stretching and working the whole of the spine, the back and shoulders, and pretty much working the whole of the body. But you are balancing on the pelvic area with one hip.

Now remember, there is a heart energy through the pelvis (tertiary connection). You are stretching forward, opening chest, and flooding heart with oxygen-rich blood. It has a lot to do with self doing the loving, and the biggest energy perhaps is self-doubt.

You second guess yourself, you doubt your capability and creativity. It comes from the negative ego or monkey mind. No doubt!

You often doubt yourself when you try to be perfect and fail. Doubting yourself is punishing yourself for failure. When confusion is pushed down inside you, it manifests as self-doubt and then transforms into fear if ignored. Learn that your doubts can be used to clear your head, re-assess, and create new ideas, inventions, changes, and dreams.

DOUBT IS A FORM OF DEFENSE

The most important thing is to question your doubts and know where they are coming from. Realise that doubt is a way of keeping you in your comfort zone. Doubt can be used as a form of defence to keep people away from you, not allowing yourself to trust anyone. Those who have a lot of doubt will always have to prove themselves by being super-achievers. These are usually the biggest doubters and are never happy with their life because of the doubt they hide within.

"DOUBT YOUR DOUBTS"
- PATRICK DESPLACE -

A prominent way people deal with their doubt is to seek a higher authority, one who can bolster their position and serve as a source of external power instead of trusting in their own inner knowing. They only have to believe in the higher authority to do it for them. This is enough.

Doubt fatigues you and drains you of your energy. Often you doubt your ability to love and maintain goodness. Which of your memories are you holding on to that are maintaining self-doubt? Doubt is a lack of trust and supports the monkey mind. Doubt is a way of avoiding being responsible.

Develop trust and self-confidence and take ownership for your actions and respond. The monkey mind says it is too simple, so doubt it, because the program is. "It must be

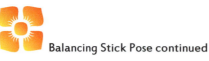

WHEN DOUBT IS REMOVED ANYTHING IS POSSIBLE.
- PAUL G BALCH -

complicated to be worthwhile." Being a cynic is one who is a doubter and who wants to look smart by challenging everything, although they often don't have the resolve to work through the situation and come to a resolution.

You not only need to love yourself, but you also need to allow others to love you. Be willing to receive love from your world. Gratitude is a very powerful energy that opens the gates to allowing more life force and opportunities to flow into your life. Being grateful is not just saying "thank you"—it relates to making the most of the gifts you have received and the greatest gift of all is LIFE. So to demonstrate gratitude for the gift of life means to live life to the fullest. This means that you make the most of your opportunities and ensure the outcome is better than expected.

ALLOW OTHERS TO LOVE YOU!

What is love? Love is the most powerful force in the universe and it helps to "pull you out of the delusion of separation" (Paul G. Balch). Most people have a type of feel good experience with someone they call their partner, so they love them. This is determined on how they perform and respond, and when they change their behaviour, love quickly goes out of the door. That love is really an addiction to a feel good emotion and will quite likely have a short life span. Perhaps that is the reason why we have around 70 percent failures in marriage today, as the foundations of the relationships are not based on solid factors. Lust is not love, yet it can be mistaken for its counterpart.

THE GREATEST GIFT IS LIFE...

Physical pleasure nurtures and can heal and restore you. Eventually you need to lift the state of pleasure into a state of joy beyond just physical pleasure. Enjoyment stretches you and challenges you to feel beyond what you know. You need to have a passion for life, a fire in your belly, and an eagerness to feel and experience more in your life.

A passion in your heart allows your soul to express itself through everything you do. Forgive yourself for your mistakes and for the hurt you have caused or allowed to happen. Forgiving yourself for all the reasons that you think you can't be fully loved is essential to create beyond what you know. Then let the love in. You are naturally built to experience bliss. It is natural, so let go of the fixation with pain and struggle . . . and fly.

Working your thighs helps to release anger. Although your thighs may burn and you may feel challenged, endure the discomfort and release the karma or blockage. We were taught by a Buddhist nun that if we pull out of a posture because it is burning, we are not releasing

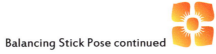
anything. If anything, we need to breathe through the burn and gain the full benefit.

Remember, when you push your knees together, you are generating magnetism. It is magnetic people who attract the right job, partner, and experience to themselves. Work on your magnetism! Apart from relieving menstrual cramping, this posture helps to balance emotional sensitivity. Many of us are really sensitive, and although this can be helpful and a great gift, it can also be a double-edged sword and we can withdraw from the public, dislike people, and appear to have little confidence. If sensitivity is managed and matured, it can be harnessed as intuition and used with psychic abilities but allows the person to be centred and secure.

"TRANSPARENT YOGI'S HAVE NO THING TO HIDE"
- JAYLEE B -

HEALING CONSIDERATIONS:

FEEL YOUR FEELINGS AND LET GO OF SELF-DOUBT

OPEN YOUR HEART AND AWAKEN NEW ASPIRATIONS

INTENSITY IS WHAT THE SOUL IS LOOKING FOR

RELEASE FEAR AROUND GIVING AND RECEIVING INTIMACY

RELEASE THE DOUBTS YOU HAVE ABSORBED

RELEASE YOUR INSECURITIES AROUND PLEASURE

STRENGTHEN YOUR INTENT AND GO FOR YOUR DREAMS

TAKE THE JOURNEY FROM YOUR MIND TO YOUR HEART

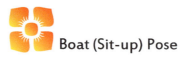 Boat (Sit-up) Pose

Padanavasana

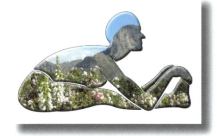

When you engage the core muscles in your stomach, you activate the Solar Plexus chakra and also activate the Kundalini chakra. When you grab your toes, forehead to the knees, you are engaging the core muscles in your stomach and lower abdomen, increasing core strength and personal power.

LADIES PUT THEIR 'RACE FACE' ON...

This posture relates to "breaking through facades and projecting false personas." Ladies put the "race face," aka makeup, on in the morning and then go out to meet the world—that is projecting a persona. People go out to a club, wearing their best dress, shirt, wallet, high heels, or cuff links and with fluffed feathers, so to speak, wanting to be noticed. When you attract another on that level, you are attracting each other on false pretences because unless you are like that in everyday life, you are not being yourself.

By not being yourself, it is a false projection. Six months later, you are not the person they originally met; you are not partying anymore. You are accused of being complacent and you may feel that you have got the relationship so you don't have to do all those things anymore. "I don't have to court my partner anymore; I can just fall back to what I normally do." You wonder why you don't see the love, feel the love, and hear the love anymore?

In the beginning you try all means to show your love. You show your love, and your partner feels your love, smells it, hears it, and gains a five-sensory experience of your love. If your main preference is to see it demonstrated and your partner likes to feel it through touch, conflict can arise if needs are not being met. In the beginning, you show it, say it, and do it.

TAKE THE CAP OFF!

But when you get complacent, you fall back to your main pattern and you only show it in your default way. For example, you only SAY "I love you" and neglect showing it physically through touch and demonstration. The other partner needs to FEEL it, because it is their main modality. What you give or show is normally what you want. It is your natural way of expression—it is what you relate to . If you like to hear love, a person can be doing everything else and you will not be able to receive what they are offering.

Most people project a false persona to hide behind. You have to play roles to fit in but

you are not trying to hide behind them; it is only for different environments so that you can

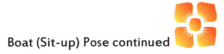
get along with others. An air force friend of ours, wearing the officers' cap and demanding what he wanted, instructing people for his needs to be met and never asking, took his energy home and expected his home environment and family to follow suit. He never took his officers' cap off and eventually his relationship broke. You need to play roles but don't get caught hiding behind them. You are much more than your persona or mask!

1 Excerpts from Unlimited Power – Anthony Robbins

"I AM A LITTLE PENCIL
IN THE HAND OF A
WRITING GOD WHO IS
SENDING A LOVE
LETTER TO THE
WORLD."
~ MOTHER TERESA -

HEALING CONSIDERATIONS:

INCREASE YOUR PERSONAL POWER

BREAK THROUGH FACADES AND PERSONAS

STRENGTHEN YOUR CORE IDENTITY

RELEASE THE FEAR OF BEING VULNERABLE

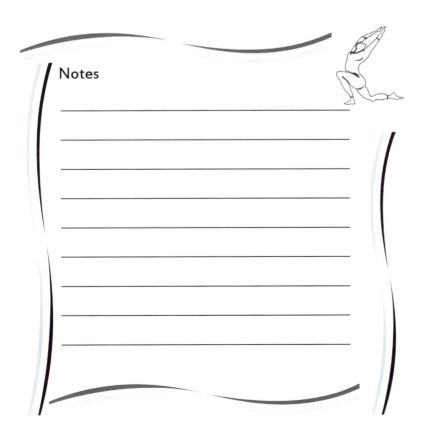

Notes

_____

_____

_____

_____

_____

_____

_____

_____

_____

You can divide people in the world into three categories:

The first category is the people who make it happen.

The second category is those who watch it happen.

The third category is those people who wonder what the hell happened.

It's up to you which category you want to fall into.

There are people who think they can and people who think they can't: They are both right!

—Henry Ford

"As a man/woman thinks, so is he/she"—is that not the familiar quote from the Holy Book? Our thoughts are the pilots of our whole being. Where our thoughts go, our bodies and emotions follow.

If you move your mind—you will change your feelings!

In general, a person is a bag of chemicals trapped within a watertight skin . . . or are they? What makes us different from each other? The exterior attributes of skin colour, hair type, age, features, height, and language, or is there something more definable that determines who we are? What makes us the same as each other? Our four limbs, head, torso and organs, habits, addictions, routines, and expectations, or is there something more definable that determines who we are? It is in our experience that each person wants to be special but working with the two options above limits our expression. To our knowledge, from a spiritual perspective, specialness is an egoic state whereby a person seeks to be regarded as above or separate from others, by way of an external feature, experience, or ability.

We prefer to embrace uniqueness and dissolve specialness. They are two very different energies altogether! Uniqueness neither separates nor elevates; it simply recognises individual strengths and weaknesses and celebrates their existence. As we do healing work with many types of people, after a time, their backgrounds all seem to be similar. Their stories carry parallel outcomes and only the "where" and "when" seems to differ. To the person who has been mugged, it feels as if they are the only person it has happened to and often they seek to use this—good or bad—to their benefit. They seek to gain sympathy, guilt, pity, money, love, and attention.

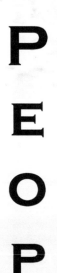

To us, their stories are the same; only their names and their individual experiences differ. The specialness lies in the belief that they are the only ones it has happened to in their world. It is difficult for them to imagine thousands, if not millions, have gone through the same. From murder, illness, trauma, rape, abuse, abduction, hijacking, betrayal, stalking, assassination, abandonment, poverty, and loneliness to richness, talents, abilities, experiences, opportunities, creations, and status—they have all been done before.

So what makes us unique? Where can we truly be regarded, cherished, and celebrated for who we are, when someone else in the world has done what we've done and got what we've got? The answer does not lie in what we have got, experienced, or achieved but in what we have done with it.

We met an incredible man one day—he was a quadriplegic (experienced many times before by others) and he had the attitude that he was alive, he had created his condition, and he wanted no pity. He wanted to be honoured for his mind, respected for his attitude, and valued for what he could bring to the table. In essence, he was not his body, he was so much more! His friends were people who celebrated his spirit, listened to his wisdom, and only helped his body where it was absolutely necessary. He was truly unique unfoldment of godliness. Most people, with perfect or functioning bodies, think that they are their bodies and nothing more—the quadriplegic has more to offer the world than them.

THE AUTONOMIC NERVOUS SYSTEM IS DIVIDED INTO THE SYMPATHETIC SYSTEM, WHICH IS OFTEN IDENTIFIED WITH THE FIGHT-OR-FLIGHT RESPONSE, AND THE PARASYMPATHETIC, WHICH IS IDENTIFIED WITH WHAT'S BEEN CALLED THE RELAXATION RESPONSE. WHEN YOU DO YOGA - THE DEEP BREATHING, THE STRETCHING, THE MOVEMENTS THAT RELEASE MUSCLE TENSION, THE RELAXED FOCUS ON BEING PRESENT IN YOUR BODY - YOU INITIATE A PROCESS THAT TURNS THE FIGHT-OR-FLIGHT SYSTEM OFF AND THE RELAXATION RESPONSE ON. THAT HAS A DRAMATIC EFFECT ON THE BODY. THE HEARTBEAT SLOWS, RESPIRATION DECREASES, BLOOD PRESSURE DECREASES. THE BODY SEIZES THIS CHANCE TO TURN ON THE HEALING MECHANISMS. ~RICHARD FAULDS

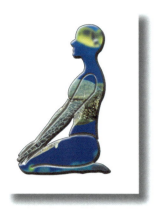

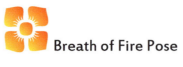 Breath of Fire Pose

Kapalbati

About fifty-thousand-plus thoughts invade our heads every day. How many of those are actually ours? Have you ever considered that? When we travel in dense traffic conditions and we sense an accident or rage rears its head inside and we feel frustration welling up, are these really our thoughts? Kapalbati Breathing is the final act of releasing all those energies and emotions that have worked their way through our system whilst we have done our yoga class. Breathing in this way is a final surrender before we lie down and enter a quiet space of acceptance or meditation.

Kapalbati breathing releases physical, emotional, and mental toxins and gives us an opportunity to find clarity. The physical toxins are released as you breathe. Many don't breathe deep enough, thereby creating a build-up of CO_2 within the bottom of their lungs, slowly poisoning themselves over many years. So there maybe some leftover CO_2 in your lungs and it needs to be cleared. The emotional centre, being the Solar Plexus, relates to the stomach, which is used in this pose, and through using your diaphragm you are working the Solar Plexus chakra. Many emotions that had become trapped in your everyday life have been released through the postures and this working of the emotional centre assists in releasing any emotional energy that is still present. The mental release comes through the intention when practicing this posture, focusing on releasing any negative thoughts on the out breath. Clarity leads to harmony and sobriety, in which we can feel free to be ourselves.

With the release of all those toxins, your energies are free and you have access to more energy for the rest of the day. It energises you. After this, lie back in Savasana and with a clear mind, image or focus on what you want. The Kundalini energy has been activated throughout the class and your energy is clear, so choose what dream you want to energise.

HEALING CONSIDERATIONS:

LET GO OF TOXIC FEELINGS AND THOUGHTS

LET GO OF ALL ATTACHMENTS TO THE PAST

FOCUS ON CREATING YOUR REALITY

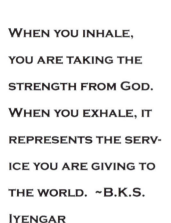

WHEN YOU INHALE, YOU ARE TAKING THE STRENGTH FROM GOD. WHEN YOU EXHALE, IT REPRESENTS THE SERVICE YOU ARE GIVING TO THE WORLD. ~B.K.S. IYENGAR

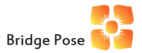

Bridge Pose

Setubanda Sarvangasana

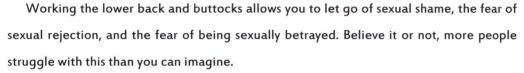

This posture is similar, in some ways, to Standing Bow Pulling Pose in the way it works the

pelvic area, the legs, and the thighs. It also works the spine, arms, and shoulders and throat area. It is an inversion posture, which allows more blood to flow to the head, activating the upper two chakras, i.e., the Forehead and Crown Centres.

Working the lower back and buttocks allows you to let go of sexual shame, the fear of sexual rejection, and the fear of being sexually betrayed. Believe it or not, more people struggle with this than you can imagine.

Having the fear that you will lose your partner to someone else focuses your love on insecurity. This type of belief is based on a lack of communication and openness with your partner. Spiritually speaking—for centuries, women have been sold on the slave blocks as young pubescent girls or discarded during the midlife period. Most of these women had no place to go to be safe and no way to feed themselves and had to take up prostitution or begging.

Our cells and DNA have recorded this, and an automatic response to being discarded is activated when women reach the midlife stage. Unless women actually deal with this and conquer it, it remains a subconscious program within.

This can lead to sexual shame, which means you feel you are not enough for your partner and sometimes this belief can lead people to believe that bringing in another person can "fill the gap"—so to speak. When you have two people in a relationship, a synergy and energy is created between the two people. A synergy means that the end result is greater than the sum of the parts. A third person has a huge impact upon you and your relationship. This applies to people wanting a child to help bring their relationship together, but if there are some issues in the relationship, bringing a third person in will exaggerate them exponentially.

Remember: Shame has a positive purpose, and that is to help you have an understanding that you have impact. The genuine feelings of remorse are experienced because your impact created hurt for someone. It can be what you did or didn't do that created the hurt, and thus you feel shame.

Another aspect of relationships that creates shame is rejection, and this creates a lot

REMEMBER: SEXUALITY IS A FORM OF COMMUNICATION IN A RELATIONSHIP...

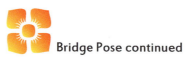 Bridge Pose continued

of pressure and fear. The fear of rejection can make someone impotent to respond and/or become aggressive, forcing something to happen. This creates a feeling of not being good enough and you can end up having to be a perfectionist to prove to the world you are good enough and to earn the right to keep your relationship, although never believing it yourself because you are never perfect enough.

You can become very needy and want to hold on to your partner and find it difficult to function alone. You need to work on having a relationship with yourself that is not based upon having to be with anyone or how others feel about you.

HEALING CONSIDERATIONS:

RELEASE REJECTION FROM PARTNERS
RELEASE INSECURITIES AROUND PLEASING YOUR PARTNER
CELEBRATE THE "TWO" OF YOU
LEARN TO HAVE REMORSE AND FORGIVE
RELEASE FEELINGS OF ABANDONMENT
LEARN TO BE CONTENT WITH YOUR GENDER

Notes

_____

_____

_____

_____

_____

_____

_____

_____

_____

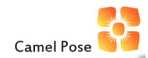

Camel Pose

Ustrasana

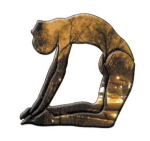

This posture releases the fear of expressing your true self and allowing the real true self to emerge. Most of our lives, we have been conditioned to respond, react, and act in a certain way. This programming has forged a mask, which we use to hide behind all the time, eventually forgetting who we really are. Most people don't even know that they wear a mask, although a few have managed to transcend it through much effort.

It is important to understand what you have become so you can let that part of you go to reclaim who you really are instead. Your true self or core identity was slowly tucked away through early childhood programming. Often as children we had to create a shield to protect ourselves from the negativity and emotional chaos that was around us, and as we become adults, this shield is no longer needed. This shield was necessary for you to survive through childhood, but it is now holding you back from revealing the real you and living life to the fullest. As you open your heart, you come to the realisation that you have nothing to hide; all of your past situations are forgiven, as you didn't know any better at the time.

Opening the heart takes courage and persistence. Often, people choose to open themselves up to feel more deeply, but as soon as a challenge presents itself, they shut down again. It is time to break through the fear of being vulnerable and allow yourself to really feel with intensity. Remember: The heart cannot lie; it is the duality of the mind and a brain with split hemispheres that can easily confuse you and cause you to be a double-minded and perplexed person in life.

Sexual addictions come in all forms and shapes and can be a source of threat and discomfort. Most people don't connect fully and utilize the energy generated through the sexual experience productively. People become addicted to the pleasurable physical feelings of sexual encounters, often neglecting the other aspects of self—being the emotional, mental, and spiritual self, thus creating imbalances. Much of our programming has come from our upbringing, and this often shuts down the sexual centre in early childhood. When parents treat a female child differently than a male child, this can create confusion and is based upon a judgement that one is better or less than the other. Parental attitudes and comments towards children, relating to sexual jokes, sexual projections, and beliefs towards sexuality, greatly influence the children. This type of behaviour manifests blockages

MOST POWERFUL POSTURE FOR EXPRESSION...

ALLOW YOURSELF TO FEEL WITH INTENSITY...

...SEXUAL ADDICTIONS...

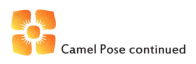

and creates challenges for these individuals to enjoy a full sexual life and explore their creativity on all levels. Release and neutralize sexual addictions and the fear around surrendering to the intimacy of sexual love. Many people will not expose what they really feel or think because they are judging themselves. When you come from a true space of love you have nothing to hide; you simply stand there in your power and reveal who you are in confidence and self-acceptance. When doing the backbend, it is enough to have your hands on your lower back without dropping them down to your feet. Most practitioners think that they must go to the fullest expression in their posture. This is an attitude that can promote injury. It is a strong backbend that triggers the Kundalini/root energy to go up the spine. It is one of the most powerful postures, as it helps to peel away the layers. This posture opens the pelvic area for sexual and creative expression, opening the solar plexus area for emotional expression, the heart centre for love and intimacy, the throat centre for communication and expression, and the centre for intuition and expressing the spiritual side of you.

**ALLOW YOUR
AUTHENTIC SELF
TO COME FORWARD...**

This posture has a lot to do with being vulnerable. The energy moving up spine breaks through fear and insecurity and allows the real you to come forward; the sexual, creative, sensitive, emotional, loving, intuitive, and expressive part of you. Focus on releasing your shyness and remember that the energy moving up the spine can cause you to feel dizzy or spin out. This is normal, as the life force of the Kundalini is reaching your brain to awaken some of the 93 percent of the circuits that have been dormant. When you touch your hands to your feet, you are releasing sexual addictions, addictions to pain and suffering, and addictions to emotional dramas, which involve being a victim or a tyrant. If you are caught up in any of those, this is posture to focus on.

HEALING CONSIDERATIONS:

RELEASE THE FEAR OF BEING EXPOSED TO REVEAL YOUR TRUE SELF

TAKE MORE RESPONSIBILITY FOR YOUR SELF

EXPRESS YOUR TRUE SELF

HELP ELIMINATE THE TOXIC NEGATIVE THOUGHTS THAT YOU
HAVE TOWARDS YOURSELF

RELEASE THE FEAR AROUND BEING SEXUALLY AND
EMOTIONALLY VULNERABLE

YOU ARE GOOD ENOUGH—FEEL GOOD ENOUGH

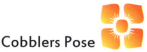

Cobblers Pose

Baddha konasana

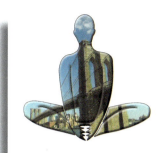

This posture helps to release rigid sexual boundaries. These can be created through your upbringing, the way you were treated when you were a child regarding being a little girl or boy. Emotional projections often are in the form of a joke, e.g., "He will grow up to be a stud and have lots of girls, he should stop playing with his genitals otherwise they will fall off, won't the boys like to get into her pants when she grows up, and I'll need a shotgun when she grows older."

Parents are not taught to be respectful towards their offspring no matter what their age is. What a parent mutters behind closed doors about a child is as detrimental as if it were directly to his or her face. Not all communication is verbal—children pick up nuances, vibrations, and attitudes. They are far more open and aware than we give them credit for.

Most emphasis is placed on mental development throughout the formative years, while the body and emotions are chaotic and there is a disregard of the sexual urges that are starting in a young person's life. This is also manifested through the more mainstream spiritual organisations, where the natural urge for procreation to take place at the right time and for the right reason is seen as a sin unless you are in a married relationship. This makes people who feel sexual and are not in a marriage feel guilty. This has had a major impact upon people regarding their sexuality. The mainstream spiritual organisations created strict guidelines around sexuality, because sexuality is a very powerful energy that can empower people and set them free, as it lifts the person into a state of bliss.

It is very difficult to stop people from having sex. The mainstream spiritual organisations have tried to control sexual expression through creating rigid boundaries around why, when, where, and with whom. The dangers are: When you allow yourself to totally be lead by this energy, and you cannot have sex for whatever reason, you could lose the impetus or reason to live. This happens.

The mainstream spiritual organisations have a great responsibility for the confusion around sexuality; people are ashamed, feeling guilty, dirty, and sinful for a natural act of expressing, communicating, and sharing themselves in a sacred way with one another.

Have respect and be willing to express and explore to get to know yourself. When you

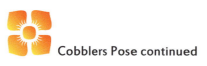

are in love and spiritually connected to the person you are sexually connecting with the creation of a baby will manifest a child of a much higher level of consciousness.

Marriage is often a burden, and for many they feel trapped rather than free to celebrate the relationship to the fullest. True matrimony means freedom and the maturity to allow the other to grow in respect and faithfulness.

Healing Considerations:

Release sexual rigidity
Sexual grounding and releasing fantasies
Create a flexible attitude towards sexuality

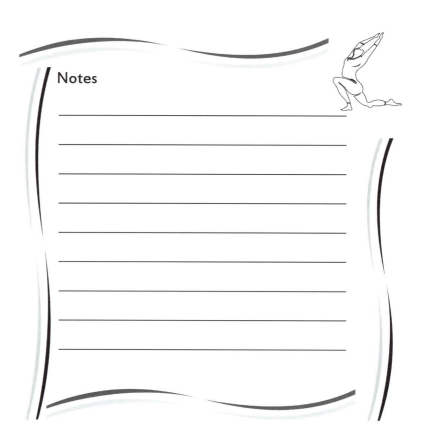

Notes

_____

_____

_____

_____

_____

_____

_____

_____

_____

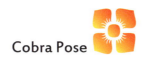
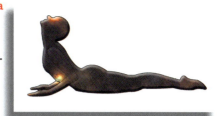

Cobra Pose breaks through self-pity and false expectations and releases insecurity, especially around manifesting.

By feeling symbiotic guilt (in other words, how can we have when others don't?), we end up feeling sorry for those who have incarnated into a more challenging reality than ourselves, and through doing so, we feel guilty for having what we have created. This relates to self-pity. We have pity for someone in a less fortunate position because we would not like to be there, so to alleviate that feeling of self-pity within us, we respond by helping or saving someone. The biggest thing is to be caring and at the same time respect the life lessons chosen by that soul.

ACHIEVEMENT ALLOWS US TO BRING SUCCESS INTO ACTUALITY
- PAUL G BALCH -

Achievement is an energy that liberates us and allows us to bring success into actuality. By celebrating achievements, we give ourselves a firsthand experience of success, giving our subconscious mind the message that we want more success in our lives. Futuristically, we can always remember and draw on that experience again to create another achievement. How often or not do we really micro-manage our failures and skim past our successes? They deserve the same considerations. It is difficult to celebrate when you are feeling guilty for what you have. You need to celebrate what you have learnt from the experience and then let it go.

HAVE NO EXPECTATIONS...

The next aspect that you need to release is the need to harbour secrets—you have to use some of your energy to continually hide a part of your life that you feel ashamed of. When you forgive and come from your heart, you will have nothing to hide about yourself. Forgive yourself, forgive the other people involved, and move on.

And then you have shame, which is associated with things you've done and thought, including the shame of existing because you were a "mistake" from birth. So many of us were not planned from the beginning, so we feel that we are a mistake. We were either a welcomed surprise or a regret for having a pleasurable time once long ago. This condition can lead to feelings of not having a place in this world or the license to live life fully. Feeling unforgivable also produces shame and sabotage as well as a feeling of undeserving.

Break down the patterns and addictions around emotional blackmail. Emotional black-

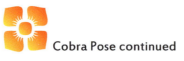

mail relates to either allowing yourself to be manipulated or manipulating on an emotional level. Creating emotional dramas to get attention is feeding on another's energy and often playing these types of behaviours rob us of our energy. It's a give/take, win/lose situation where we either forfeit some of our energy to another in the drama or we take their energy from them. Either way, true discipline teaches us to manage our own energy and not to get caught up in any drama!

Society's expectations trap many of us. What society projects onto us is a set of do's and don'ts. We need to function in the world, although the barrage of expectations we often receive can create emotional baggage that can become so heavy that our creative selves are stifled, our dreams squashed, and our real selves buried.

This is a back strengthening posture and it takes a lot of effort, so do not hang out! The lower back in this posture relates to releasing issues with self-pity. Self-pity tends to affect the Sacro-Iliac area. Self-pity is a lack of self-love and can dehabilitate anyone who gets caught feeling sorry for themselves.

The lower back also relates to issues around abundance and the fear of creating. If you recognise that you have this fear, set your intention to release these fears before class and forget about them. As you go into the posture, control your breath and know that you are moving these issues out by doing this posture.

You place a lot of expectations upon yourself and you can develop a curvature in your spine. Release those expectations. The Master Enlightened Master told us that "expectation freezes the potential of the future to ONLY WHAT YOU EXPECT. If you get any more than what you expect then you have created a miracle." Have no expectations! Allow yourself to be amazed and don't limit your dreams!

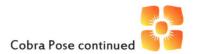

HEALING CONSIDERATIONS:

RELEASE YOUR FEARS AROUND SECURITY AND ABUNDANCE

RELEASE THE FEAR OF LOSING WHAT YOU HAVE CREATED

LET GO OF SELF-PITY AND GET ON WITH IT!

AWAKEN EMOTIONAL VULNERABILITY AND HONESTY

AWAKEN TRUE RESPONSIBILITY AND RESPOND IN THE MOMENT; DON'T WAIT!

RELEASE SOCIETY'S FALSE EXPECTATIONS

RELEASE SELF-PITY AND TAKING YOURSELF TOO SERIOUSLY

RELEASE THE NEED TO USE EMOTIONAL BLACKMAIL

RELEASE THE NEED TO CREATE EMOTIONAL DRAMAS

YOGA IS THE PERFECT OPPORTUNITY TO BE CURIOUS ABOUT WHO YOU ARE.
~JASON CRANDELL -

Notes

_____

_____

_____

_____

_____

_____

_____

_____

_____

S T R E S S

It is commonly and scientifically understood that stress kills people, affecting them physically, emotionally, mentally, and spiritually. You have two systems, the sympathetic and parasympathetic nervous systems. They work antagonistically like the bicep and tricep muscles in your upper arm. The parasympathetic nervous system is what operates in your everyday life; however, if you experience a challenge where you feel stress, you shift to the sympathetic nervous system. Once the stressful situation disappears and the challenge is over, you will automatically shift back to functioning from the parasympathetic nervous system. You need this balance to survive. If, however, you are always functioning from the sympathetic nervous system (running on nervous energy, and being addicted to stress as a motivating force in your life) you will start to burn yourself out. If you are operating at this level and another challenge manifests you may end up losing control and cracking up.

When you are under tremendous stress and anxiety, the first thing that will happen is that your thyroid stops functioning; it shuts down. Because of that it either becomes a hyperthyroid—trying to work despite the fact—or a hypothyroid, giving up and not working. When your thyroid stops functioning, your thymus gland collapses and your adrenal glands start working for themselves as well as for the thyroid. You then begin to function on your adrenals.

To do that, the adrenals release not only adrenaline but also cortisol. It is the body's natural production of artificial cortisone. It is anaesthetic in its nature and is a steroid. The cortisol numbs the pain in the body and creates a false sense of calm and being in charge. It is damaging to the body because it eats away at the heart, liver, and pancreas—the three major organs of the body.

It also does damage to the brain in the neurotransmission of information. It is not enough that you would notice it any one day, but over time it will shorten your life. Your liver has to work overtime, so it drains the glucose from your blood, therefore you get low blood sugar reactions, and in women it causes what we call oestrogen dumps. This is where all of a sudden the hormones of the body, in response to the glucose being pulled out of your blood, will dump oestrogen and that level of oestrogen is damaging. Even now doctors are discovering that levels of oestrogen can produce cancer. This can also happen in men.

With our relaxation meditation exercise, your level of stress will eventually be brought right down to a deep-sleep level within twenty-one days. Your stress levels will naturally pick up a little as you go about your everyday life, although you will feel more relaxed after each session and over the next three weeks it will gradually lessen. Unless you reach your inner core of calmness, it is difficult to tap into your full potential and access the higher intelligence and the hidden resources of your mind.

There are no mistakes in life, only opportunities to learn something more and new. If you go through and complete the whole process, you will completely break through your old paradigms and your life will become an amazing adventure. You will be far more conscious, and well on your way to becoming the master of your own destiny. It is time to consciously write, direct, and live your own dreams.

Practical exercises addressing STRESS:

Exercise: Write down the five main specific triggers that manifest stress in your life.

Exercise: Research where stress becomes a positive motivator to prompt you into action.

Exercise: Look at how often you let yourself down by not following through.

Exercise: Write down where you felt you made mistakes in your past. Admit them, take ownership of them, and see what that situation was teaching you.

Exercise: Write down five main experiences where you have allowed people to interfere and sabotage your plans and dreams in life. Take ownership and realize how you allowed this to happen.

Exercise: Write down where you are giving your energy and authority away to others.

'YOU CAN CHOOSE TO MOVE BEYOND MOANING, GROANING, BITCHING AND COMPLAINING. THE PAYOFF IS PERSONAL INSIGHT, INTEGRITY AND THE FREEDOM TO DO BETTER'
- MAUREEN DAIGLE-WEAVER - (A PERSONAL FRIEND)

ABLE TASMAN NATIONAL PARK - NEW ZEALAND

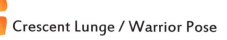

Crescent Lunge / Warrior Pose

Virabhadrasana

This posture is very similar to a Triangle Pose combined with a Camel Pose. You are expressing and balancing the higher aspects of your inner male and inner female. This inner male is known as the Animus and the inner female is known as the Anima.

The male energy relates to willingness and action. The masculine gives permission to take action, sets a direction, and responds. It constantly works on creating structure, seeking meaning and understanding, and the state of doing—DO IT! The female energy is the feeling of emotion and desire behind the action. Being feminine is nurturing and open to be nurtured, giving and receiving, the power and essence behind the action, the creativity and the love, allowing the expression of intuition and perception, balancing, and the state of being—BE IT!

TAKING ACTION IS A MALE ENERGY...

When these are in balance, they create a sustaining impact that keeps going on its own momentum. This has to be done and expressed through love, and this posture opens your heart to allow that. Crescent Lunge or Warrior Pose is about expressing the true inner self in a balanced way and allowing it to shine through to the outside world. Balance your personal inner ideal image of a man and woman and the outer relationship to the males and females in your life. Many fall in love with their perfect image of the Anima or Animus and then cannot experience a full relationship with someone in their life because they cannot ever match the perfect image within.

THE POWER BEHIND THE ACTION IS A FEMALE ENERGY...

Look at where you have tried to take action in your life and fallen flat on your face because you lacked substance and preparation (power behind). And look at where you felt you could take action and make a difference, but you couldn't or wouldn't respond and therefore procrastinated (ability to take action). This is very much the armchair critic, who could do better than everyone else but has never take action to show what he/she is made of.

You may have heard that behind every successful man is a powerful woman. You need a powerful feminine energy behind your action to be successful, man or woman.

Having an active masculinity and powerful femininity is needed to create; the goddess and the god unite for manifestation and creation to take place. It does not matter whether you are by yourself, accessing the Male and Female within, or in a relationship or even a same-sex relationship—one partner will supply the feminine energy and the other will supply the masculine for the relationship to manifest and create a synergy of growth that can be sustained.

MOUNTAIN POSE TEACHES US, LITERALLY, HOW TO STAND ON OUR OWN TWO FEET…. TEACHING US TO ROOT OURSELVES INTO THE EARTH…. OUR BODIES BECOME A CONNECTION BETWEEN HEAVEN AND EARTH.
~CAROL KRUCOFF

HEALING CONSIDERATIONS:

TAKE ACTION WHEN IT IS NECESSARY

EXPRESS HOW YOU REALLY FEEL

BALANCE YOUR INNER MALE AND INNER FEMALE

WARRIOR POSE ALLOWS US TO BATTLE INNER WEAKNESS AND

HELPS US TO FOCUS.

Notes

_____

_____

_____

_____

_____

_____

_____

_____

_____

_____

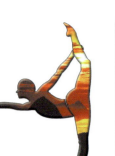

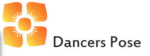

Dancers Pose

Dandayamana Dhanurasana

You may feel it in your buttocks, hips, thigh, lower back, and wrists. When you start bringing your body down, parallel to the floor, it is working deeply into your lower back, and whenever you do a back bend, you trigger Kundalini energy up the spine. It is working tremendously through the pelvic area. Dancer's Pose releases shame and shame builds up around the buttocks, and every single person needs to deal with it. When you are blamed for something you are not responsible for, it is internalised and you can feel flawed. When parents project on to you to be the best, because it makes the parents feel validated, they project this on to the children and it results in shame. Absent parents can manifest a type of shame and can cause conflict later on in life.

As we grow up, we end up experiencing shame on some level or another. As early as eighteen to thirty-six months old we start feeling shame. When you started to express your-self and you were told "no," it made you feel there was something wrong with you. If you suppressed it, it became an embarrassment and you felt that you were not allowed to make a mistake and that you were a mistake. It also happens between six to eight years old when you push away from your mother and connect more with your father.

Then around the age of twelve years, you push away from your father and connect with your world. The separation creates shame within you. The chemistry of your body is altered through shame; this internally alters your brain development and functioning. You may have been taught by your perfect parents that you were flawed, defective, and not as good as them, or your parents were less than perfect and taught you to be defective and flawed as a way of life.

You may have felt shame through divorce or death as well as creating a feeling of not being good enough. You were always being put down. In many ways, we have abandoned our true nature and ourselves, and it is time to respond to the call of your soul and be true to yourself again. If you create a strong relationship with yourself, you will never feel aban-doned. We betray ourselves often by not being ourselves and we feel we need to fulfil the expectations of others to be good enough and feel accepted and the need to belong.

"WE ARE LIKE LITTLE FOUNTAINS RISING UP FROM THE DEEP, UNDERGROUND RIVER OF GOD."
~ UNKNOWN -

OUR PARENTS MIRROR OUR SELF WORTH AND SELF LOVE...

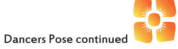

Movement around the hip rotators is releasing betrayal and abandonment. Abandonment is when someone promises to be there for you and doesn't turn up or when your partner doesn't turn up on time or has a greater commitment to work than to you.

You have heard and perhaps often felt the fear of being successful. Most people say they are afraid of failing, although they may feel unhappy in continuous struggle. They are so used to this state of life that it has become their comfort zone, and to really succeed would mean that they have nothing to complain about and no one to blame anymore. So for most people it is the fear of success and then having to keep it up that scares them, not failure.

You need to be yourself and remember that sex is a sacred way of expressing yourself with another, from all levels of your being. An enlightened Master once said that when you have sex with someone, you exchange soul energy and carry the energy of that person and the encounter for the next seven years. It is wise to be very selective about who you sexually connect with and what space are they in when you do connect. Sexual expression needs to be multidimensional, beyond just the physical body, as many people feel wanted physically and are then left feeling unsatisfied. To really feel sexually loved is to connect on all levels when having a sexual encounter, where your partner respects you and there is no pretence or expectation involved.

Two points in the front of the groin (either side of the pubic region), with the opening of the hips, release the need to flirt to get attention. Remember, when you flirt, you are receiving energy from others, but what type of energy are you receiving? It is not necessarily the type of energy you want for yourself: Their thoughts, attitudes, emotions, and perceptions can be polluted. Love yourself enough that you go within to find the energy that you want; it is the purest source!

The first sexual interaction you ever had is energetically encoded in your DNA for life and it gets passed down to your children . Remember, the soul records ALL your first-time experiences! So, have fun and have as many NEW experiences as you can, from the small to the wondrous. Allow the energy of the soul to guide you on an amazing journey through life.

"...YOU ARE NOURISHING SOMETHING THAT'S VERY IMPORTANT — YOUR DREAMS."
PAULO COEHLO

PEOPLE FEAR SUCCESS MORE THAN FAILURE

BE SELECTIVE WITH YOUR SEXUAL ENCOUNTERS

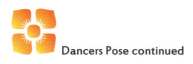

Dancers Pose continued

I WANT MY INNER TRUTH
TO BE THE PLUMB LINE
FOR THE CHOICES I
MAKE ABOUT MY LIFE –
ABOUT THE WORK THAT
I DO AND HOW I DO IT,
ABOUT THE RELATION-
SHIPS I ENTER INTO AND
HOW I CONDUCT THEM.
- PARKER J. PALMER

HEALING CONSIDERATIONS:

EXPRESS AND RELEASE SEXUAL SHAME

RELEASE THE FEAR OF ABANDONMENT AND BETRAYAL

BE WILLING TO RECEIVE SEXUAL LOVE

RELEASE THE NEED TO FLIRT SEXUALLY

BALANCE YOUR MALE AND FEMALE ENERGIES

DEAL WITH IMAGE ISSUES

[2] Anastasia – by Vladimir Megre – Ringing Cedars Press

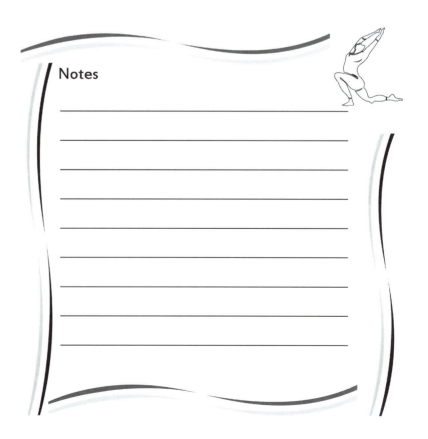

Notes

_____

_____

_____

_____

_____

_____

_____

_____

_____

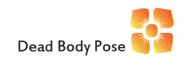

Dead Body Pose

Savasana

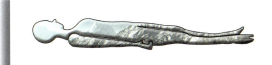

This posture is a very challenging one for everyone, as you need to allow your mind to shut off and move into a true meditative state beyond normal thinking. You cannot force yourself to stop thinking; you focus your mind on entering a state of stillness then allow yourself to enter it. It is all about surrender. It is the allowing that is the tricky part for most. Many teachers ask their students to focus on their breath to get out of their heads. This works, although you can get caught up in watching your breath, which can become a distraction into entering the higher states of consciousness beyond thought. So the best way to enter a space where there is no thought is through surrender.

A dead body does not think on the physical level, as the spirit has left the body and this is what this posture is about. Shift beyond your physical body and attachments to the physical world. In meditative states you learn to drop your attachment to your physical body and also your mind, as the mind is a tool for your soul and consciousness and the mind is not you and you are not your mind. This state, if performed correctly, helps your thoughts and feelings to become balanced. It can awaken a new sense of imagination, desire, and mental determination when returning to the present. Basically, it sharpens your mind and it is like refreshing your computer software.

Meditation is, at the beginning, a state of mind where you eventually go beyond the mind. If you enter this state fully, you will have no pulse and your breathing will have stopped, as you will have stepped out of your body and will be operating at a higher level of consciousness. This is the whole aim of spiritual studies and disciplines and where you start to step on the path of true mastery.

> CORPSE POSE RE-
> STORES LIFE.
> DEAD PARTS OF YOUR
> BEING FALL AWAY,
> THE GHOSTS ARE
> RELEASED.
> ~TERRI GUILLEMETS -

HEALING CONSIDERATIONS:

LEARN TO DROP THE ATTACHMENT TO YOUR BODY AND MIND

RELEASE THE TENSION IN YOUR BODY

CREATE STILLNESS OF MIND AND BODY

LEARN THAT THE TRUE STATE OF MEDITATION IS "NO MIND"

BELIEFS

Beliefs are the foundation of our lives and outlooks. We gather them, unhindered, from our parents, peers, friends, schooling, and circumstances. We all get the basic program to survive this world, but sometimes survival is just not enough.

A good sculptor will choose a piece of rock and carve away at the rock to form a figure of his choosing. A great sculptor will choose a piece of rock, see an image in the rock, and begin to remove what doesn't belong until the image is revealed in all its glory. Each human being receives a set of beliefs to help them to survive as a "rock in potential." Within each human is a potential masterpiece, but the pieces that don't belong need to be removed piece by piece.

We are supposed to grow up and begin the process of contemplation, whereby we sift through the morass of beliefs we have absorbed and we choose which no longer suit us or reflect accurately who we are. Most never begin that journey into their lives and change their beliefs. They settle for who they are and what they have and the beliefs that they have taken on. They don't question and challenge—mostly, they assume that they cannot change what has been done and said.

On the contrary, a change of attitude is enough to change a belief and reveal a wonderful countenance. Remember: Your attitudes, thoughts, feelings, decisions, and choices all depend upon your beliefs. It is hard work, chipping away at the beliefs and letting them go, because often they remind us of someone we once cared for. Realise that your backgrounds and circumstances may have influenced what you have become, but you are responsible for who you are, and your view of the world depends upon how much you love yourself, respect yourself, and trust yourself.

To change our beliefs, we need to work on our thoughts: Your train of thought is important because it determines your day, your experiences, and your reality. Thoughts know no boundaries, so they travel through walls, beyond borders, and into minds. They can enter the tiniest crack in a mind that knows no love and change its destiny, so do not brush your thoughts off as if they are nothing or are never heard because they are in your head. They are heard; if not by anyone else, they are heard by yourself.

Change your choices and responses—a person who is brought up in a conservative family may make choices that limit freedom and do not explore reality or take any chances, believing they are unsafe or risky. But a person who is brought up in a family with little boundaries may make choices that shy away from limitation, commitment, and engagement, believing they are claustrophobic.

Always seek to question!

Practical exercises addressing BELIEFS:

Exercise: Sit and contemplate various topics that carry strong beliefs, not only for yourself but in your world. For example: your faith or lack of it, political view, beliefs around sexuality, gender roles, children, and marriage.

Exercise: Now, consider why you believe what you believe using the topics above. Are they beliefs that you have previously examined and made your mind up about or are they passed from your family, friends, and the media or books you have read?

Exercise: If you have encountered a belief or beliefs that you don't want anymore, begin by making new choices and decisions and change that self-image and the way you see yourself.

KEEP YOUR BELIEFS POSITIVE BECAUSE
YOUR BELIEFS BECOME YOUR THOUGHTS
YOUR THOUGHTS BECOME YOUR WORDS
YOUR WORDS BECOME YOUR ACTIONS
YOUR ACTIONS BECOME YOUR HABITS
YOUR HABITS BECOME YOUR VALUES
YOUR VALUES BECOME YOUR DESTINY!
- MAHATMA GANDHI -

ABLE TASMAN NATIONAL PARK - NEW ZEALAND

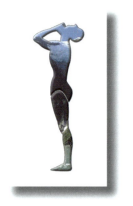

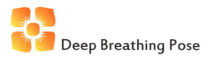

Deep Breathing Pose

Pranayama

By default, we tend to take on other people's responsibilities, which really have nothing to do with us. Yes, we can assist people in life, although it is not for us to take on their burdens—especially those close to us, which often happens. In a nutshell, we try to do so much for others and end up neglecting ourselves. It is essential that we look at our own motives for doing so. Is it simply, trying to be a saviour or being a martyr, needing external validation so that you can feel better about yourself, and/or trying to impress others to win their favour? Which one?

STOP HOLDING BACK...

When it comes to holding back sexually, often we are thinking far too much about our everyday life when being intimate with a loved one in a sexual encounter. This thinking becomes a distraction to being able to surrender to the experience and blocks our ability to go all the way and really open up and be ourselves. This relates to control issues and having a difficulty in letting go and achieving climax.

THERE ARE NO MISTAKES...

Fifty percent of people were conceived without planning and careful thought! Unknown to most, this can have a huge impact on you, in a way where you feel you don't have a right to exist, always apologise for yourself, and have a fear that you don't really know yourself and are not being yourself. So, you were not a MISTAKE! There are no mistakes under the sun . . .

We were offering a seminar in Seattle when we were introduced to a bar manager of a friends sports bar and gave him a flyer of one of our seminars. It stated that "You need to know yourself to find yourself," to which he wryly replied, "If I found myself I wouldn't know what to do with myself."

STOP PROCRASTINATING

It is important to be willing to receive feedback from your environment no matter what type it is. This allows you to know the impact you are having in your world and then you can evaluate if you are on track or need to change your approach. The challenge comes when the feedback is not what you like, so your ego tries to use this information to diminish your self-esteem and self-worth. It is very important not to put off until tomorrow what can be achieved today. Far too often we become lazy and fall into procrastination, which robs us of the ability to create our dreams.

84

Procrastination is a slow way of dying and giving up on life and having your own dreams. Many who procrastinate end up becoming the harshest critics and feel they could have done better, but never deliver because they don't have what it takes to respond and make a difference. It is often a way of not taking ownership of what is happening in your life. You ARE good enough!

YOGA DOESN'T TAKE TIME, IT GIVES TIME.
~GANGA WHITE -

HEALING CONSIDERATIONS:

RELEASE AND EXPRESS THE BURDENS OF OTHERS

RELEASE SEXUAL INDECISION AND THE INABILITY TO SURRENDER

NEUTRALIZE INDECISION AND PROCRASTINATION

RELEASE THE FEAR AND CONCERN AROUND MAKING MISTAKES

BE COMFORTABLE WITH EXPRESSING AND RECEIVING FEEDBACK

Notes

_____

_____

_____

_____

_____

_____

_____

_____

_____

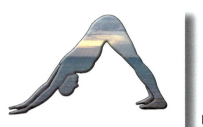

Downward Facing Dog Pose

Adho Mukha Savanasana

Feel it in your heels, ankles, wrists, legs, shoulders, spine, and brain as you move into and through Downward Facing Dog Pose. It's the perfect moment to let go of projecting a certain image in which you need to feel in control. Let go of living up to your family's projections and expectations!

AFTER 21 YEARS OF AGE, YOU NEED TO PARENT YOURSELF...

Once you reach the age of twenty-one, it is time for you to start living your own life and parenting yourself. Many parents want to keep telling their children what to do with their lives, and in some cases live their lives for them and even through them. They want their children to achieve what they didn't and give their children opportunities that they didn't have, with no consultation with what their children want to do with their life. You can receive guidance from your family, but once you have turned twenty-one, it is time for you to make your own decisions about life and be the adult, parenting yourself. Parents, allow your children to be adults. Be their friend instead, and you may find that your relationship will reach a whole new level altogether! Don't allow others to manipulate you into doing things that you may not want to do. It is easy to go along with what others want when you want to keep the peace, but then you give up your free will and allow others to control you.

LIFE CAN BE A GRAND UNFOLDING JOURNEY...

Control can take place in the following ways:

1. Threat—"Do this or else you will have to pay a big price."

2. Emotional blackmail—"How can you do that to me after all I have done for you?"

3. Rational—"Let's talk this through and be logical and reasonable."

4. Manipulation—"Stay with me and I will promise I will reward you."

Let go of your inflexibility about having fun. Fun is a very important thing in life. Enjoyment allows one to have a light heart and you spot these types of people from a mile away. They are a pleasure to be around. So focus on having more fun with those around you, especially family. You need to be more flexible about being creative with your humour. Expect nothing and then everything is a miracle because you end up getting more than what you expect and life is a grand, unfolding journey.

LAUGHTER, IT IS SAID,
IS A TRANQUILIZER
WITH NO SIDE EFFECTS,
SO TAKE TIME OUT TO
SMILE!
- UNKNOWN -

HEALING CONSIDERATIONS:

HAVE A NEW OUTLOOK ON LIFE

LEARN TO PARENT YOURSELF AND BECOME INDIVIDUAL

LET GO OF BEING EMOTIONALLY BLACKMAILED AND MANIPULATED

FOLLOW YOUR HEART AND UNFOLD YOUR OWN DESTINY

HAVE FUN—NUMBER ONE MANDATE FOR LIFE!

Notes

_____

_____

_____

_____

_____

_____

_____

_____

_____

T I M E   M A N A G E M E N T

Have you ever wondered why you and a colleague have a different concept of time? You both work in the same office, doing similar jobs, yet one of you feels the day went fast and the other feels the day went slowly. How is that possible?

Time is a state of mind and can be changed at will. It is a choice and an attitude. We have regularly given ourselves the suggestion each night and each evening that the hours we are at work will go fast and the hours we are at home will go slowly. We experience the effect every day of our conscious choice to make time work for us and not have time dictate to us.

On some occasions, we have actually arrived at our destination in miraculous time. That was our attitude. In a world that is frantic with production times, deadlines, traffic, and the feeling of no time, we often find ourselves losing control and our stress levels climb higher each moment. Take time to catch your breath and relax. That moment could be the difference between life or death, sale or no sale, calmness or worry.

Tasks: Each evening you will write down three tasks that you will complete the next day at exactly the designated time. You need to complete this process for twenty-eight days consecutively. This means eighty-four tasks in a row over four weeks. This exercise creates a clear connection between your conscious mind and your subconscious mind. By programming an instruction the night before, you then carry out the task the next day.

You will learn about time management and about the relationship you have with yourself. What is important is that you keep the tasks and your progress to yourself, so you don't disperse your energy and become influenced by the opinions and agendas of those around you. Many who have completed this exercise have ended up missing the next task by being distracted.

After you have completed your tasks for twenty-eight days, you may tell the world. You need to write down your tasks of each day to come and you will see everything fall into place elegantly. You have trained your subconscious mind to achieve the targets and strengthened the connection between the conscious and subconscious minds.

Become aware of how you operate on autopilot in most situations. You tend to become a creature of habit, by switching off and not being present while going about your daily life. I remember visiting one of my mentors many years ago. I was still in the frame of mind where I was at the feet of the guru waiting for something profound to be passed on to me.

He told me that it was time to start tying my shoelaces differently. I was not sure if he was joking, although he seemed serious, so I went to apply this exercise. I became far more conscious about living life and making decisions. I am far more aware of what is happening around me at all times and I am always looking for new ways of doing things.

This process really opens up your mind and keeps it sharp and fresh. From now on shower, dress, eat, and tie your shoelaces differently. Apply this to your life and the way you drive to work. You have to be more conscious to know what you're doing and consciously choose.

Practical exercises addressing TIME MANAGEMENT:

Exercise 1: Evaluate and write down what percentage of the time you dwell on negative outcomes.

Exercise 2: Become conscious of focusing on constructive thoughts from now on.

Exercise 3: Ask yourself how often you follow through on tasks that you have set for yourself.

CASSOWARY BIRD - AUSTRALIA

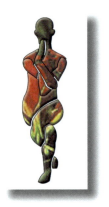

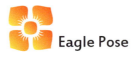

Eagle Pose

Garudasana

According to a Tibetan Lama we have worked with for many years, judgement is a major obstacle for most people. Yoga helps to the burn away at a cellular level the judgements you have held on to and the emotions you have not released in your life. This allows new energy to be made available for your use in more constructive areas.

EAGLE WORKS ALL THE MAJOR JOINTS IN THE BODY...

Judgement is what holds us back from communion with our God selves and the Supreme Being. We need to connect with our true self and go beyond judgement. Every experience is an opportunity to learn, and according to your preferences, your attitudes and beliefs determine what you learn. What you learn is good because life is a mirror and it is all about growth. As you judge another, you trap a part of yourself through your attachment at that level of thinking and your energy at that moment of judgement, thus you can become trapped in the past. It is far too easy for people to worship, judge, and criticize than to actually learn to think and apply the knowledge they have learnt so far.

In life if you feel stiff throughout your body, it is a manifestation that you are becoming rigid in your mind, because the mind impacts upon the body and the body impacts upon the mind. You can open your mind to having different viewing points. Rigid thinking taken to the extreme can manifest as arthritis and widespread bone degenerative diseases. It includes rigid thinking towards yourself and towards your world. The self is reflected in the pelvic area and the world is reflected in the shoulders. Overall, it is rigid thinking that you are releasing.

SEXUALLY WANTED IS NOT SEXUALLY LOVED...

Next step, you wrap your arms into a knot, but a lot of weight is centred around the pelvis, like in Awkward Pose, and you are pushing the thighs together. This flushes the reproductive system, while you are really stressing the I.T. Band by working the thighs—this can release perfectionism, self judgement, and rigid thinking.

Perfectionism is a static view of a potential outcome. "Life will be perfect if I can create a perfect partner, home, etc."—static outcome. If you do attain the perfect picture, it will never satisfy you. If you have a perfectionistic outlook on life, you are always going to have a lot of anger, judgement, and internal conflict because it is unattainable. Perfectionists become control freaks because no matter how much effort they put into a project, it

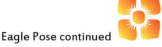

will never be good enough and their need to control the outcome is out of proportion. It doesn't matter how much energy they invest, it is not good enough.

Perfectionism alleviates or overcompensates the feeling of not being good enough. The biggest doubters are the most competitive people—they have to compete to prove themselves, to be good enough because they doubt themselves. People who want to be number one always are full of doubt. You can be number one or you can be AT ONE. When you always need to be number one, you are never at total peace and you are egoically driven.

We all have the need to feel loved, and in our relationships, we have the need to feel sexually loved and secure. Many women feel sexually wanted although, sadly, they don't feel sexually loved. Men want them for their bodies and looks and not to really connect with who they truly are. This relates to creating sexual fusion—where a synergy is formed and both partners feel more connected with a stronger bond.

Sexual fission happens when two (or more) people get together sexually and a huge release of energy happens, although the love and heart connection is missing. After this type of encounter, you end up feeling more separated and alienated. You are left asking, ,"Why did we bother?" This is a child/adolescent way of thinking about sexuality, connecting only on the surface with multiple partners because you never experience the depth of intimacy and synergy with fission. Many stay here at this level of sexual encounters because they are afraid of intimacy and commitment. When you respect the inner identity of the person you are connecting with and you are open to all levels of expression (physical, emotional, mental, and spiritual) you can surrender to the experience of expressing with the whole self that you are to another. This relates to creating sexual fusion—where a synergy is formed and both partners feel more connected with a stronger bond during and after the encounter.

A DASH OF COURAGE AND A TEASPOON OF WILLINGNESS...

One of the most important spiritual tasks to master this lifetime is to feel secure in creating, celebrating, giving, and receiving pleasure and fun on all levels. When dealing with the fear of change (relating to the kidneys), you tend to try to manage and maintain what you have, out of fear. Stepping out of our comfort zones can be terrifying; however, a dash of courage and a teaspoon of willingness to change always go a long way. We all can have magnificent amounts of potential that is yearning to be expressed. Imagine that each person has a part of the Supreme Being inside, which wants to be seen—just a little bit of awareness and self-development is needed . . .

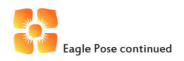

EVERBODY MAKES MIS-
TAKES, THATS WHY
THEY PUT ERASERS ON
THE END OF PENCILS
- UNKNOWN -

HEALING CONSIDERATIONS:

LET GO OF RIGID THINKING AND RELEASE PERFECTIONISM

RELEASE SELF-IMPORTANCE AND THE NEED TO BE BETTER THAN OTHER PEOPLE

RELEASE SELF JUDGEMENT AND SOCIETY'S JUDGEMENT

AWAKEN CREATIVITY AND THE CELEBRATION OF LIFE

RELY ON YOURSELF AND LEARN TO TRUST YOURSELF

HAVE DIFFERENT IDEAS ON THE WORLD AROUND YOU

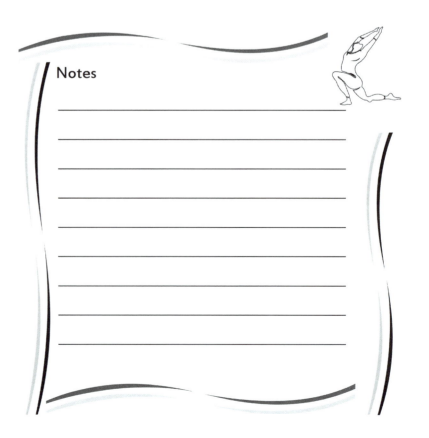

Notes

_____

_____

_____

_____

_____

_____

_____

_____

_____

_____

Fixed Firm Pose

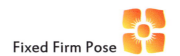

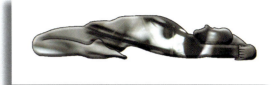

Working deeply into ankles (Sacral), calves (solar Plexus), knees (Heart), thighs (Throat), and lower back (Sacral), you are releasing a lot of energies in this posture. Frustration, in general, manifests in front of the calves—and sexual (Sacral Centre) frustration.

Working deep in the knees, you are releasing sexual resentment. Allow yourself to receive sexual love. There is a difference between lust and love and you should know the difference. Sexual love includes tenderness, caring, intimacy, and fulfilment. Let go of sexual resentment; it can be a soul-destroying blockage. This takes place when your needs are not being met and most of the time you are not communicating your needs to your partner. Sexual pleasure is allowed! Many people we have worked with have a fear of receiving pleasure. They don't allow anyone to spoil them or pamper them, treat them or surprise them. You are worthy and good enough.

ALLOW YOURSELF TO BE PLEASURED...

Your dream needs to evolve and keep growing, in such a way that your dream can operate on its own and keep growing. When you become a parent, your life revolves around your children. You give up your life, you don't have a life anymore, and you are a mum or dad now. When your children leave home one day, what are you then, without them? Children should fit into your life, not you fit into your children's life!

You take yourself too seriously! How you look, how you speak, what others think of you, if you are good enough, are you aging, and many more pressures are placed upon yourself. It is time for you to relax about yourself and learn to laugh about YOU! When people make jokes, laugh. When friends tease you, laugh. The world will be a better place. When you place most things into perspective, they will not matter a week later; they will have been forgotten, so why take them too seriously in the first place?

CHARITY BEGINS AT HOME...

Create emotional stability and security in your life by loving yourself first and then loving others. If you fill your cup constantly until it is overflowing, then everyone around you will gain from that overflow. However, if you are constantly giving and you never fill your own cup, eventually you find you have none to give and you are left wanting. When you learn to love yourself, very little can steal your peace. Centre your "home" within and be at peace.

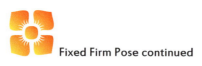

"EVERYTHING CAN BE TAKEN AWAY FROM A MAN BUT ONE THING: THE LAST OF THE HUMAN FREEDOMS – TO CHOOSE ONE'S ATTITUDE IN ANY GIVEN SET OF CIRCUMSTANCES, TO CHOOSE ONE'S OWN WAY."

~ VIKTOR FRANKL -

HEALING CONSIDERATIONS:

LET GO OF TAKING YOURSELF TOO SERIOUSLY

FOCUS ON STABILITY AND SECURITY IN YOUR EMOTIONAL INTERACTIONS

ALLOW YOURSELF TO BE SEXUALLY LOVED

FLUSH OUT HEAVY EMOTIONS ALLOW YOUR DREAMS TO MANIFEST AND EVOLVE

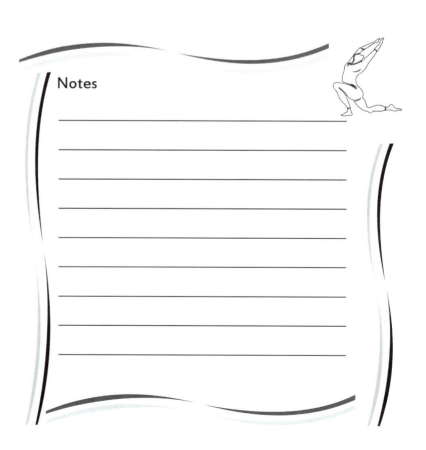

Notes

_____

_____

_____

_____

_____

_____

_____

_____

_____

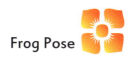

Frog Pose

Bhekasana

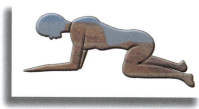

Frog pose releases your inner expression and sexual expression. Taking a look at the pose, we can see that the hips and ankles are worked really hard as well as the knees. There is an opening in the pelvic region and the Sacral Centre is activated. Express your own needs instead of going along with the needs of others and putting their needs first.

We can get caught up in what the other person wants, even to the extent that we will do things that we would not normally do. This happens when we get caught up in someone else's agendas. You need to express your own needs and preferences. Your needs are the things you have, to feel secure, and your preferences are what you would like to have. Are your needs being met or are your preferences being met?

ARE CAUGHT IN ANOTHER PERSON'S DREAM?

Take a look where you are getting caught up in other people's dreams. It is much easier to be a follower than a leader, but you end up being caught up in someone else's dream. This happens through the way we are educated and through our careers. Often when we need acceptance, we tend to do what others want, to create a feeling of fitting in and belonging. We bite our tongues and do not express what we are really feeling, so that we don't rock the boat and create waves. We often do this through the fear of being rejected. Often in life we are creating someone else's dream through our work, through trying to please our partners, family, and friends. It takes courage and self-belief to create our own dreams.

This can manifest as working for yourself and setting goals and plans for your future, instead of just living day to day and being a cog in the wheel of someone else's dream. Of course not everyone will have their own dream, because they have the dream of their parents, of their partners, of their corporations, etc. While this does serve a purpose, they are not free.

I remember a friend saying, that to have a J.O.B. means JUST OVER BROKE and most jobs will not pay you enough to set yourself up to be free to do what you want in your life. They offer you security and stability at the cost of giving up your freedom, being free, and creating for yourself.

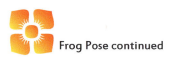

Frog Pose continued

Yoga is the practice of quieting the mind. ~Patanjali, translated from Sanskrit

Many often hold back from expressing what is in their heart for the fear of being judged or rejected, but you need to express it no matter what and you will find those who really respect who you are and love you for being you will celebrate you. Instead of looking for permission from others to go for your creative ideas, give yourself permission and go for it.

Healing considerations:

Express yourself sexually and naturally
Have your own dream and create what you want
Express what is your heart and be true to yourself
Speak your truth!

Notes

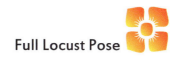
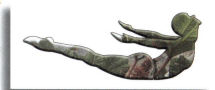

In Full Locust, you are working through self-sabotage and shame, as one of the strongest energies being released. You are breaking through being motivated out of concern, fear, and necessity. Necessity and opportunity are the opposite of each other. Although necessity is the "Mother of All Inventions," it does not leave much window for elegance. Focus on the opportunity in life and respond when it knocks. When opportunity comes your way, you first receive a whisper, then when that is ignored, you receive a shout and finally, you get a scream.

The whisper may be a little argument, a shout is a full-blown fight, and the scream is when your partner throws in the towel and walks out. The whisper is elegant and subtle; it is the quiet knock of the spirit. When you have a dream, it is elegant, easy, and graceful. Reassess! When are you leaving things to the last moment? What are you refusing to hear or take heed of? Don't put things off! The energy of necessity connects with fear and concern, and so the outcome is mediocre. If you respond to the energy of opportunity, it is amazing and fantastic. Break through that energy. When an opportunity comes up, take the chance, otherwise the energy that has built up for it can diminish and you lose out.

You are here to express all aspects of yourself constructively and impeccably. This posture helps you release fear around expression. You need to express your power, and this is done through taking responsibility, which is being able to choose the optimum response and responding, feeling secure and stable. It also relates to expressing your creativity as well.

WHEN OPPORTUNITY KNOCKS THE FIRST TIME, GRAB IT AND HOLD ON...

HEALING CONSIDERATIONS:

LISTEN TO THE WHISPERS
CHANGE THE NEED TO LEAVE THINGS TO THE LAST MINUTE
CHECK YOUR CONCERN GAUGE—DO THINGS YOU LOVE TO DO
REWARDS FOLLOW OPPORTUNITIES—SEIZE THE DAY!

Understanding the ego and its roles is essential in your understanding yourself. As the ego is a part of you, you come to the realisation that you need to transform your ego from foe to friend, as it is an important part of your make-up.

Now, in most people, the ego has become altered and negative. Having an ego, the human race has become the most powerful being on the planet, but the way we have worked with the ego has made us very weak. An important thing to realise that you cannot kill your altered/negative ego; you need to transform it to work with you and not against you. It is like a knife; it can be used for good or left alone it could be used as a weapon.

The ego's role was to inform us of what is happening in our world, making it possible for us to be aware and in touch. When we refused to receive/respond and take ownership of the incoming information, the ego ended up with the responsibility by default and this has turned it negative, as it was never designed to be in charge. Now the altered/negative ego has taken over interpreting the incoming information, but also the outgoing response, giving meaning to everything that is happening in your outside world and the internal world of our minds.

This is the constant voice within your head that is very controlling, judgemental, critical, and manipulative, telling you that you are the worst or better than everyone else. Learning to understand and transform your altered/negative ego is an essential task in your spiritual development. This will determine whether you gain freedom and unleash your true spirit or you stay managing a mediocre life like most. Remember, you have free will and you can say to the voice within you "thanks but no thanks" and change the internal message to one that is positive and constructive. It takes discipline but the benefits are well worth it.

I owned a Formula One prototype two-stroke racing motorbike—a one-of-a-kind machine. One morning on the weekend, I was going for a joy ride when I remembered I had an appointment with a friend. I took a shortcut through some backstreet's in the suburbs to connect with a major road (three lanes each way) to return to my home. As I approached the intersection, I saw a car a way off and the rest of the road was relatively free. Remember: I had one of the fastest motorcycles registered on the road. As I pulled out to the centre lane of the road, I saw this car approaching much quicker than I anticipated. So I twisted the throttle and my front wheel came up in the air. I then changed to second and then third gear, while accelerating and still on the back wheel. I was trying to keep an eye on this car bearing down on me. By the time I knew I was out of danger, I had hit 180 kilometres in a 70-kilometre zone and this car came within 10 metres of me. It was challenging, although I felt excited. As I slowed down and this guy came beside me, swearing at me, looking very angry, I laughed at him, blew him a cheeky kiss, and zoomed away.

He ended up beside me again and this time he swerved his car to push me into the median strip in the centre of the road. I then realised this guy was crazy and I needed to get out of there. So I ended up getting into a right hand turning lane only, and as he followed me I pulled out of the lane as easily as a motorbike can and left him behind. This guy, who was a total stranger, allowed my actions into his mind to upset him and he put himself and other people in danger. In other words, he allowed my actions to enter into his mind and to control his life.

Practical exercises addressing REACTIONS:

Are you allowing people to enter your mind and control you?

How are your reactions being affected by your environment?

Realize that whenever you create a judgement, you are most often diminishing or placing yourself or something else on a pedestal.

Exercise: Write down what aspects of your environment this week triggered reactive responses within you (good and bad).

Exercise: Write down what aspects within yourself triggered responses within you (good and bad)?.

"THE BEST YEARS OF YOUR LIFE ARE THE ONES
IN WHICH YOU DECIDE YOUR PROBLEMS ARE YOUR OWN. YOU DO NOT
BLAME THEM ON YOUR MOTHER, THE ECOLOGY OR THE PRESIDENT. YOU
REALIZE THAT YOU CONTROL YOUR OWN DESTINY." ~ ALBERT ELLIS -

BLUE CRANE - NATIONAL BIRD OF SOUTH AFRICA

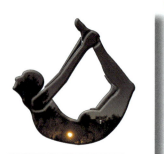

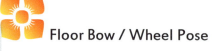

Floor Bow / Wheel Pose

Dhanurasana

There is a very powerful Kundalini release in this posture, deep into the lower back, and this is where a blockage is released, relating back to the age between three to seven years. Hands are connecting around the feet, opening up the front side of the pelvic area, and the activated Kundalini Energy first reaches the Sacral Centre, where sexual insecurities and blockages can be released. During the ages of three to seven, something called the Oedipus complex can take place, where parents working and educating their children project a joke or judgement on to the children.

As another example: When small children first begins to discover themselves, their first explorations are through touch, and the initial sensations can cause the children to find enjoyment in themselves. This is all part of the natural discovery of our own bodies; however, parents who are less informed may slap the child, punish them, or humiliate them in public, without thought to the impact. The sexual blockage experienced later in life can come from an experience similar to this one.

WE HAVE TREMENDOUS IMPACT ON OUR CHILDREN IN THEIR FORMATIVE YEARS...

Laudosis is a strong curvature of the lower spine and is often associated with an energetic blockage that is known as the Castration Syndrome, experienced very young in life. It can stem from emotional abuse, sexual innuendos, physical abuse, sexual abuse, or mental abuse. If a little boy is urinating in the lounge into a pot plant whilst there are visitors, often the parents, out of humiliation, will slap the child, and later in life he may find it difficult to urinate in public places in urinals. We have a tremendous impact on our children.

THOSE WHO CRITICIZE OUR GENERATION, FORGET WHO RAISED IT!
- UNKNOWN -

The fear of letting go is often linked with control issues, and this is where people hold back and don't relax. It is so important to be able to simply let go, to maintain healthy lifestyles. You need to put the clutch in regarding life and in take time to reassess and get in touch with where you are, how you feel, and where you want to go regarding your life. It is essential to let go and take time out regularly to really be in touch with life.

Those who criticize our generation forget who raised it!—Unknown

Many have a fear of reaching their goals and being successful. The fear of success is because you are much more used to failure; although it is not what you would prefer consciously, it is what you know, and success creates fear because it is what you don't know. The strong backbend impacts the kidneys—so this posture releases the fear around change and rocking the boat. Many people fear change because they cannot exactly predict the outcome, so they can become paralysed. Fear stops the life force from flowing naturally up the spine, so this posture helps to move the energy up the spine. The fear of responsibility is a big one for many because of their programming when they were young. Responsibility was a dirty word because when something went wrong their parents asked who was responsible for the trouble. This type of impact then created an association between responsibility/blame/guilt, and therefore influencing many not to take responsibility for their lives. Responsibility is the ability to respond and to choose the best response.

Breaking through the need for external validation is essential, as this can leave you at the mercy of your those around you and you will do whatever it takes to feel you are good enough. This means putting yourself last and looking after others' needs first, and often you end up feeling left out and not appreciated afterwards.

In Conjunction With: (Wheel) Upward Bow Pose—Urdhva Dhanurasana

This posture is similar to Floor Bow, except with this posture you are also following the curvature of the earth and therefore resonating to earth energy, which grounds you. This assists in releasing fear on a physical level and works all chakras.

ANGER IS A CONDITION IN WHICH THE TONGUE WORKS FASTER THAN THE MIND
- UNKNOWN -

THE FEAR OF CHANGE ROCKS THE BOAT

HEALING CONSIDERATIONS:

HELP TO BREAK THROUGH FEAR
RELEASE CHILDHOOD TRAUMAS
TAKE RESPONSIBILITY FOR YOURSELF FIRST!
STRENGTHEN CONCENTRATION AND MENTAL DETERMINATION
DEVELOP INTERNAL BALANCE AND HARMONY

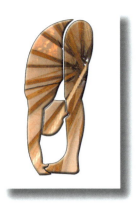

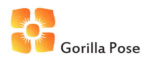

Gorilla Pose

Padahastasana

With Gorilla, we are forward bending and inverting our body so there is a shift in our perceptions relating to control and listening to the monkey mind. The monkey mind is the little voice within your head that is often constant and highly controlling. This voice is very critical, controlling, judgemental, and competitive. Most have a need to be in control; for many the fear of losing control is controlling them so they have lost control even before they start.

LET GO OF THE NEED TO MICRO-MANAGE...

To really have control of one's own life, you can let go of the need to be in control of everything in your life because you know in the blink of an eye you can be in control of it again, therefore you are not trapped in your need to be in control. You can be in control within a situation or you can try to have control of a situation; they are quite different. The first situation you only need to be in control of yourself; the second situation you need to control yourself and whoever else is involved in the situation, which takes a lot more of your time and energy, eventually draining yourself.

This can manifest as a need to micromanage everything and everyone in your life. Often this can happen with a position of authority needing to control and delegate in your work environment that then bleeds into your personal life and instead of just playing that role at work you live it as a way of life.

MONEY IS A BEAUTIFUL ENERGY

Far too often this also happens with people who have manifested wealth; they use their money to control others because of their station in life. If you want to be free all you have to do is give up everything else, and this also includes offering freedom to those who are in your life. Often we try to fight and control this voice within, and by doing so we end up giving it more energy to control ourselves.

This voice is a feedback mechanism to help you understand what is happening in your external world; where it all went astray was you didn't always want to respond to your world and the feedback so the ego was left to make the decisions and respond for you. Therefore the ego became negative as it was not ever designed to be in charge of your life. Now it wants to be in charge and in control of everything in your external and internal world, giving its own meanings to what is happening and what you should do about it. Many people feel this voice is their conscience, which is not the case.

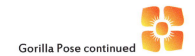
Your true conscience will never tell you what to do or distort your view of the world; it respects you too much to do that. This monkey mind voice is always telling you what to do, what is wrong, right, good, bad, that you must, you shouldn't, you can't, you have to. . . . It is very critical and controlling.

We tend to get caught up in our own mirror of self-reflection when we listen to the monkey mind too much, which for many creates an image that is based upon a competitive of having to be either better than or less than someone else. When you feel insecure you tend to feel the need to control even more your outside world. This posture helps you break through the controlling effects of your internal dialogue (mental distractions). When you take yourself too seriously, you end up becoming caught in the altered ego. When you over-identified anything in life you can be controlled by it. Whether it is money, glamour, sexuality, strength, or flexibility, when this happens you end up being at the mercy with whatever you have identified yourself with and it ends up controlling you.

**IT BEGINS WITH YOUR
BELIEFS...**

This can happen with relationships, where people give away their individuality, giving everything to their partners. They end up being dependent on their partners to validate them, to feel powerful and secure. Your partner's behaviour ends up controlling your own behaviour so the relationship becomes a dance of having to control your partner's behaviour so their behaviour will not control yours. You have created a co-dependency. The other person's behaviour becomes more important than you living your life because you have made their life more important than your own. This interferes with your ability to focus and concentrate on yourself and to know what you want and need to do for yourself in life. We need to transform our relationship with this voice, thus transforming this voice from being negative to positive.

HEALING CONSIDERATIONS:

YOU CANNOT FORCE YOURSELF TO LET GO OF THE PAST

LET GO OF NEGATIVE EMOTIONS

KNOW THAT YOU CAN CREATE AND MAINTAIN ABUNDANCE

RELEASE MATERIALISTIC CONTROL AND LIMITING BELIEFS

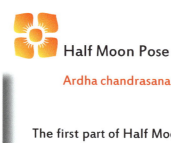

Half Moon Pose

Ardha chandrasana

The first part of Half Moon has a lot to do with the Solar Plexus Centre (emotions) and the Throat Centre (expression). Because you are working the whole torso, it has a lot to do with the expression of your self-image.

You are working up your back and two things are happening here: Your hips relate to your Private Image—how you see yourself—and your shoulders relate to your Public Image—how the world sees you. It has everything to do with bringing a balance in harmony, of the image you present to your world, and how you see yourself. For most people, it is the opposite—you project a happy, smiley face to the world, which you hide behind and hide what is really going on within you.

BALANCE YOUR PRIVATE AND PUBLIC IMAGE...

Unless you go within and discover the real you and cultivate an internal image that is authentic, most often your projection (mask) is the opposite to the way you are truly feeling or your projection is a defence mechanism. Strengthen your self-image so that you don't need the external validation from your world.

Working the hips from side to side helps to free up the stubbornness you have towards yourself. In the second bend backbend, you activate all the chakras if you go deep enough. Bending back far enough until your head drops lower than your heart will activate the Psychic and Intuitive Centres.

RELEASE YOUR FEARS AROUND 'BEING YOUR-SELF'...

Any backbends trigger Kundalini energy and it may bring up the insecurities that you have lodged deep within. Opening up the chest releases your fears around being yourself. Opening up the front of your body you are exposing yourself, and it is helping you deal with vulnerability, but by bending backwards it is exploring the unknown.

You cannot see where you are going, so it is breaking free of your comfort zones, stepping out of your normal paradigm, and exploring beyond what you know. If you step into the unknown, that is where you grow the most. If you remain in the known, you will feel very comfortable and safe and secure, but you stand a chance of stagnating and you won't grow.

In the third forward bend, you are dealing with issues of control. The hamstrings have to do with control and flexibility in the postures—by going into a posture you have the poten-

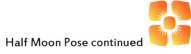
tial to release any blockages; if you are more flexible, it is an indicator that you don't have as much emotional investment in holding on to the blockage. Flexibility is NOT an indicator of the lack of blockages but it does indicate that you can release blockages in that posture easily if you so choose. If you are very stiff and tight, it is often an indicator that you have a strong investment in that issue and there is a payoff, a payoff you don't really want to give up.

To some degree, ALL OF YOU are control freaks. The more structured you are, the more planned your life is and the more inflexible you are about change—if you are too structured and planned there is no room for mystery and magic and there is no room for growth. Have loose plans!

You either control yourself to such a degree that you are not you, or you are trying to control everyone else. If you are trying to control everybody else, you may be tired and burnt out and you will find it a difficult task because you will be wasting energy continuously. Unless you have consciously observed and worked on your control issues, they are still in your life. No one is exempt!

Being that the third part of Half Moon is an inversion posture; it helps to clear the monkey mind, which likes to be in control. It is continuously telling you, you can't, you must, you shouldn't, you have to—it is the monkey mind or ego.

**NEVER MISS AN OPPORTUNITY TO MAKE OTHERS HAPPY, EVEN IF YOU HAVE TO LEAVE THEM ALONE IN ORDER TO DO IT.
~AUTHOR UNKNOWN -**

ARE YOU A CONTROL FREAK...?

HEALING CONSIDERATIONS:

RELEASE THE FEAR OF BEING FOUND OUT THAT YOU ARE A FRAUD

LET GO OF FALSE PRETENCES AND FACADES

LET GO OF OLD PAIN AND TAKING YOURSELF TOO SERIOUSLY

ALLEVIATE YOUR ANXIETY AND REDUCE YOUR MENTAL STRESS

LET GO OF FEAR AROUND FAILURE

AWAKEN YOUR INTUITION AND KNOW THYSELF

RELEASE AN OLD SELF-IMAGE

RELEASE THE FEAR OF PROJECTING YOUR TRUE SELF-IMAGE

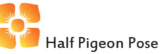

Half Pigeon Pose

Kapotasana

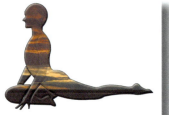

Self-importance is a major tool of the altered/negative ego and it fools you into believing that you are either better than everyone or less than everyone—you're the best or the worst. This means that most people are investing way too much of their prana (life force) into maintaining their self-image and feeling better or less than everyone else.

YOU ARE AT THE MERCY OF OTHERS...

Self importance is the feeling that you are more important than others or less important than others. When you feel more important than others you usually demand others to meet your standards and you tend to be arrogant and controlling because you think you know everything and are the best. When feeling less than, you are caught up in judging everyone to be more than you and therefore you justify manipulating everyone to get them to help you, because they are in a better position than you. You are still controlling, usually by making others feel guilty or through manipulating.

Usually people want to feel and seem important and need to bolster their lack of self-worth. There is a misconception that "loud is proud," but often Tall Poppies are pulled down by other misguided people who seek fame and fortune. When people relate to you in this way, they determine how you feel about yourself and you are at the mercy of how others see you. On the other hand, you can feel not important enough and you can allow yourself to be treated less than what is acceptable. You can end up drawing these types of people into your life to prove that you are not good enough. What is the most important thing is how you feel about yourself, independently of everyone and everything. This issue has a big impact upon people, to the extent that it utilises approximately 90 percent of people's pranas (life forces) to maintain their own importance or lack thereof.

USING ILLNESS TO MANIPULATE OTHERS...

People will even create illnesses to get others to do it for them, and this is a very powerful way of controlling and manipulating others to get what you want. This energy robs you of most of your life force and renders you impotent, which is what the negative ego wants because you are then predictable and easily controlled. It is essential to reach the point where what others think, how they behave, and their differences in no way leave you feeling less or more valuable. Honour that everyone has their own unique talents and differences and celebrate them, as this is where you learn.

It is very important that you believe in yourself and come to the realisation that you are capable of absolutely anything.

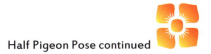

HEALING CONSIDERATIONS:

RELEASE YOUR FEELINGS OF BETTER THAN AND LESS THAN

IGNITE YOUR SELF-CONFIDENCE

ENHANCE YOUR SELF-ESTEEM

BE SELF-SUFFICIENT, RELYING ON YOURSELF

GOOD FOR THE BODY IS THE WORK OF THE BODY, AND GOOD FOR THE SOUL IS THE WORK OF THE SOUL, AND GOOD FOR EITHER IS THE WORK OF THE OTHER.

~HENRY DAVID THOREAU -

Notes

_____

_____

_____

_____

_____

_____

_____

_____

Now, Bill is a farmer living outside of a small town where he has been for many years. Bill is a very religious man and dedicated to his faith, but every ten years or so there is a huge flood in this area. The storms appear and the local river starts rising and the locals panic. The local ranger, who knows Bill personally, drives out to his farm to help him collect his important possessions with a four-wheel drive vehicle so that he can go to higher ground safely.

As the ranger arrives at Bill's farm, he is sitting on the front veranda reading his bible. The ranger asks Bill to grab his belongings and come with him. Bill replies, "I believe in my god and my god will save me, thanks but no thanks, go save someone who needs saving." The ranger then receives a call on his radio, so he has to leave. The ranger calls the police who have a boat picking up stray animals and people who become stranded. The police agree they will attempt to rescue Bill. The flood has risen and the floor of Bill's farmhouse is under water.

As they manoeuvre their boat close to his front fence, a log hits the boat so the police throw Bill a life line and yell out to him to grab it and they will pull him to safety. Bill is sitting on his table reading his bible. Bill replies, "I believe in my god and my god will save me, thanks but no thanks, go save someone who needs saving." The police then almost get overturned by debris and the current of the river and they also get a radio call so they have to leave as well.

The police call the army, who have a helicopter in the area. They ask if they can fly over and try to help Bill leave. As the helicopter arrives, the whole farmhouse is almost under water and Bill is sitting on his roof reading his bible. The helicopter pilot calls Bill on a speaker to grab the rope ladder and they will drag him through the air to safety. Bill replies, "I believe in my god and my god will save me, thanks but no thanks, go save someone who needs saving."

The helicopter then also receives a call and has to leave. The story goes that Bill drowns and moves to the other side in the soul world. When he arrives there he sees god waiting for him. Bill says to god, "I pray to you all my life and believe in you and you let me die, what type of god are you?" God replies, "I send you a four-wheel drive, I send you a boat, and I send you a helicopter and you tell them to go away. What more do you want?"

You are always are at the right place at the right time. It is up to you to be awake and sense what is unfolding in front of you. If you look at the story, the first opportunity was more elegant for Bill as he could bring his belongings and it took little effort to hop into the four-wheel drive. The next option Bill had was to hold onto the life preserver and be dragged through the water. More challenging and less elegant.

The last option was far more challenging, being dragged through the air holding onto a rope ladder. This happens in life when you resist the opportunities, often because you cannot see what is unfolding, so you judge and refuse to respond. The next opportunity becomes more and more a necessity. Self-importance is the enemy of self-esteem and blocks intuition. Most successful people in business rely on their gut feeling and make up their mind in thirty seconds and take a long time to change it. Most people in life take a long time to make up their mind and change it in thirty seconds. Three moves of intuition come your way; the first is a whisper, the next is a shout, and the last is a scream, and this usually involves an impact on the physical body—an accident, broken bones, hospitalisation, relationship break-up, and disease all fall into the last state. Try to listen for the whispers; they are more elegant!

Practical exercises addressing INTUITION:

Exercise: Freezing a thought in your mind, sit quietly and watch your thoughts for a few seconds. Then focus upon one thought and set the intention for that thought to freeze in your mind. You become aware of this thought without engaging or interacting with it, judging, criticising, analysing, rationalising, intellectualising, or justifying. Be neutral. Simply observe it as if it were not your own. This is the first move towards a powerful, interconnected, and telepathic mind.

INHALE, AND GOD APPROACHES YOU.
HOLD THE INHALATION,
AND GOD REMAINS WITH YOU.
EXHALE, AND YOU APPROACH GOD.
HOLD THE EXHALATION,
AND SURRENDER TO GOD.
~KRISHNAMACHARYA-

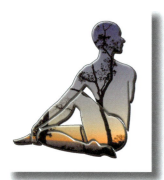

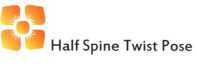

Half Spine Twist Pose

Ardha Matsyendrasana

Our self-image and self-esteem stem from our relationships with the father figure in our life. If it was a turbulent or disapproving one, then it is likely that our self-esteem may have taken a blow. Self-esteem can affect our ability to create, money issues, career choices, and myriad other areas in our life. Nothing robs us more than a disapproving father who cannot celebrate our successes as we encounter them. Our self-esteem has a lot to do with how the world sees us and how we see ourselves in the world. Recognition and self-value are generated from our self-esteem.

YOUR FATHER IS THE SOURCE OF YOUR SELF ESTEEM...

Our image is layered. How we see ourselves and how others see us are often entirely different. We encourage people to take a holiday to a destination where no one knows them, where they can present a new self-image. The people around them treat them according to the new image and this helps to reinforce it. When they return to their usual life, something has changed and they find it easier to be the new image. Most times, without reinforcement, our friends and family prefer to keep us the way we are; it makes them feel comfortable and they resist change.

Half Spine Twist Pose triggers the Kundalini energy, creating greater security and giving us more access to life force.

Because there is a spine twist, the spleen, kidneys, and adrenals are worked. The energy to release here is the FEAR OF CHANGE. Our kidneys are crucial to this and we fear change when we are entering a space of the unknown. Often people will get infections or painful kidneys when they are being prompted by their soul to change an area in their lives. Change is good. It is a space of surrender and growth. If we did not change, we would not grow and our lives would become stagnant and unfulfilling.

SURRENDER TO CHANGE!

Being creatures of habit, we like to stick with what feels comfortable and known, but often it is habit that grinds us into a hole of our own making.

Release those emotions that well up and surrender to the change that is going to take place in your life, if you so choose.

Your self-worth is most times based upon others who are important to you in environment. If a friend says it is so then we believe them, not questioning or having our own

110 thoughts. People project what they want to see and have their own agendas for those pro-

jections. If you are comfortable with who you are, then those around you should accept you. When we give our power to another, their opinion becomes more important than our own. In your world, your opinion about you is best. It is not so much what others say about you but what you say about yourself.

Self-love stems from the relationship you had with the mother figure in your life. If you received an abundance, there is a good chance that your self-love is good, but if your relationship with your mother was poor, your self-love issues manifest in several areas. One of them is the constant need to receive love from others, resulting in a co-dependency. Another is that you need others to fill your cup, as you do not know how to fill your own. Yet another manifests as an emptiness inside that you cannot fill and without self-love, you cannot truly give love to another. You have to know it to give it.

HEALING CONSIDERATIONS:

HEAL YOUR SELF-IMAGE AND SELF-ESTEEM

RELEASE THE FEAR OF CHANGE

HEAL YOUR SELF-WORTH

RELEASE YOUR STUBBORN ANGER TOWARDS YOURSELF

HEAL THE INSECURITY AROUND SELF-LOVE

I HAVE NOT FAILED!
I'VE JUST FOUND
10,000 WAYS
THAT WON'T WORK.
- CHUCKLE -

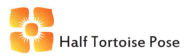

Half Tortoise Pose

Ardha Kurmasama

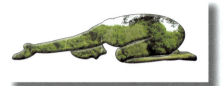

Make sure you get that forehead to the floor and you lock out those elbows. You are flattening the upper part of the back and working deep into the shoulders.

As you stretch forward core muscles are engaged with the stretch forward, but it is important for you to flatten the back. People's spines start to curve through the upper to middle part of the back when they take on too many obligations and responsibilities for others. "My job is to keep my wife happy!" It is NOT my job to keep my wife happy, it is her job. If I keep myself happy, then we have happiness to share with each other. It is not about relying on another to fill up your cup, it is your responsibility.

FOREHEAD TO THE FLOOR IS MORE IMPORTANT THAN HIPS TO THE HEELS...

Responsibility relates to the shoulders and the upper part of the scapular—focus on being more responsible for yourself than for others. Your forehead to the floor is more important than your hips on your heels. The earth is a neutral being—it does not judge. It can neutralise any negativity and garbage and internal dialogue. Clear your mind and rejuvenate and energise your mind—putting your forehead on the floor is your refresh button.

JUDGED EMOTIONS ARE LIKE A STAGNANT POND...

You can begin a makeover of your attitudes and beliefs towards pleasure and relationships. Relationships were meant to be enjoyed, bring growth, and give us an opportunity to share. I always share in seminars that, as a couple, my partner is MY opportunity to express my love in an intense way and vice versa. Cheekily, my outer female form is attracted to his outer male form AND my inner masculine is attracted to his inner feminine. It is not only about form; his qualities of caring and nurturing attract my inner qualities of decision-making and focus. Switching between gender roles can be fun if you are both open to growth.

YOUR PARTNER IS YOUR OPPORUNITY TO SHOW YOUR LOVE...

Let go of those sticky, negative emotions that trap you when you least expect it. Emotions of the past are not emotions that flow. They are stagnant and trapped, and having a continuous referral to them is like drinking stagnant pond water. When we hold on to emotions and experiences from the past, we are sending precious energy elsewhere and we are not benefitting from it in the moment. This is like driving your car down the road and constantly looking in the rear-view mirror; you will not get very far in life if you function this way. Many of our gifts are dependent on a great deal of energy being present in our current lives; if our energy is scattered in bad ordeals and memories, we do not have the energy to express our gifts and to fulfil our full potential.

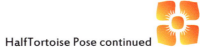

We grow up receiving the do's and don'ts from our world and we strive to fulfil each obligation, until we partially achieve or give up feeling we are failures. Examine the responsibilities you have taken on to your shoulders and determine if they are yours or they have been projected on to you. "Father is a doctor so I must be one" or "I have to uphold the family name by earning a certain salary." What do you want for yourself to be happy and fulfilled? What is expected of you as a mother or father, a daughter or son? What dreams do you have and what are you doing to realise them? Do you enjoy the sense of achievement gained from what you achieve? Are your dreams simply someone else's because you never had a dream of your own?

Don't build other people's dreams all your life. Give yourself a chance to build your own and often it is easier to start small and simple at the beginning. Don't fit your dreams into your pocket—allow your pocket to grow to meet the needs of your dreams.

Commitments can be regular bills to pay because you have agreed to pay them and they have benefit for you—a car to drive around in, furniture, water and electricity are all commitments with benefits. Obligations, however, are burdens that you have willingly taken on, whose benefits are few and far between. Decide between your commitments and obligations and make some positive decisions.

IF YOU FALL DOWN 6 TIMES, GET UP 7
- JAYLEE B -

DECIDE BETWEEN COMMITTMENTS AND OBLIGATIONS

LET YOUR POCKET GROW TO MEET YOUR DREAMS... NOT VISA VERSA!

HEALING CONSIDERATIONS:

LET GO OF PAST EMOTIONS

INCREASE THE CIRCULATION TO YOUR BRAIN

EXPRESS AND GROUND YOUR DREAMS

LET GO OF THE EXPECTATIONS OF THE WORLD

LET GO OF THE OBLIGATIONS OF THE WORLD

CLEAR YOUR THOUGHTS

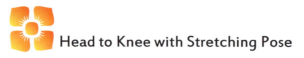

Head to Knee with Stretching Pose

Janushirasana with Paschimotthanasana

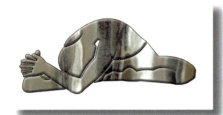

As in Standing Head to Knee Pose, this posture releases control; however, your coccyx is on the ground, so it not so much about self-control, but about controlling influences towards relationships. Your right side relates to your masculinity, thought, action, and doing—the left side relates to femininity, emotions, receiving, and being. As you relax into the pose, head to knee on the left-hand side, you begin to release the need to control and judge the females in your life, and on the right-hand side, you release the need to control and judge the males in your life. (There is usually a chuckle in the class when we mention this.) This posture also releases judgement towards females (left) and males (right). Kicking the heel out releases chauvinism, which is trapped in the back of the calves.

CHAUVINISM IS JUDGING ONE GENDER TO BETTER THAN THE OTHER...

What is chauvinism? Chauvinism is judging the feminine energy to be superior to that of masculinity or masculinity to be superior to femininity. It is embodied in many ways, which most know such as: judging men to be better than women, extreme feminism, and in more elusive ways, valuing your mind over your heart, mental development over emotional development, IQ but no EQ, and thinking your feelings instead of feeling your feelings.

TEACH YOUR CHILDREN TO CREATE FOR THEMSELVES...

Focus on freedom—for you to be free, allow the people in your life freedom. It is a difficult challenge being a parent with children. Help your children, who are largely egocentric, to understand the accountability of freedom. They should know the difference between right and wrong and the discernment to choose with a healthy conscience, rather than simply because they have been told to make the choice, because it is what their mother or father want. Stop playing the role of being parent when they need to parent themselves. It is absurd that parents break their backs, creating an empire for their children, when they should be teaching them to create for themselves.

YOGA IS A GIFT TO THOSE WILLING TO RECEIVE IT...

The double leg stretch out in front, with fingers wrapped around the big toes, has lot to do with controlling yourself too closely and taking yourself too seriously—have more fun. We all get caught trying to control our experiences, relationships, and environment. It is often a self-preserving mechanism and seldom does us any good. Because of control (excessive) we lose out on moments of surprise, unknown experiences, and joy.

Once again, let go of the control in relationships and surrender. Be willing to trust and allow the other person to surprise you. Trust is a good energy, but so much happens in our lives that we don't trust anyone, especially ourselves. We doubt our choices and then doubt our partners, because they are part of the choices we have made or we have allowed. Give someone else the benefit of the doubt and surrender the iron-clad control.

Releasing emotions allows us the experience of "dying to the different energies that had been trapped within our physical and emotional bodies." Often "dying" to an experience or emotion leaves us feeling lost and slightly off course. As with all types of death, a period of "mourning" or readjustment needs to take place, and perhaps alone time. If you have had a big release (crying or simply screaming into a pillow), be alone—be All One.

Access the full extent of your life force and be centred. Yoga is a gift and only a small part of healing is the physical posture. How we approach the posture, what we are thinking about, and our internal dialogue all play a part in healing during the class. Being centred allows you to access abundant life forces and absorb value from all your experiences. You have experiences so that your soul can know and can feel.

Integrating yourself into your world is sometimes challenging. You see things and you experience things, but you are never taught emotional discipline as a child. Most people, emotionally, are trapped somewhere in their inner child, whilst their intellect is trapped in their adolescent and their physical bodies have become adult. Most adults revert to the emotional patterns they expressed in their childhood when pushed into a tight corner. We are taught to deal with physical things through sport and intellectual things through school, but no one ever offered a class in dealing with emotions.

We have judged our emotions and worked very hard to hide the unsavoury ones from our world and to our own detriment. Stuffing them down into our bodies has caused more harm than we can imagine. Yoga is a constructive and safe way in which we get to release and learn from those trapped emotions. We stress that love is like a rubber ball, which can be bounced now and then, but trust is like a crystal ball. Once dropped, it shatters.

THE FIRST AND GREATEST VICTORY IS TO CONQUER YOURSELF; TO BE CONQUERED BY YOURSELF IS OF ALL THINGS MOST SHAMEFUL AND VILE.
~PLATO -

SURRENDER THE IRON-CLAD CONTROL...

LOVE IS LIKE A RUBBER BALL...

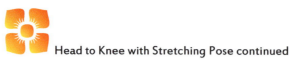

HEALING CONSIDERATIONS:

RELEASE CONTROL ISSUES AND JUDGEMENTS IN RELATIONSHIPS

DIE TO THE PAST AND LET GO OF TRAPPED EMOTIONS

ACCESS THE FULL EXTENT OF YOUR LIFE FORCE AND BE CENTRED

ABSORB VALUE FROM ALL YOUR EXPERIENCES

RECOGNISE THAT YOU ARE A "FEELING" BEING

DON'T HIDE YOUR EMOTIONS, DEAL WITH THEM, DON'T DENY THEM

RELEASE CHAUVINISM—WE ARE ALL GODLY

WHETHER YOU THINK YOU CAN OR THINK YOU CAN'T, YOU'RE RIGHT.
- HENRY FORD -

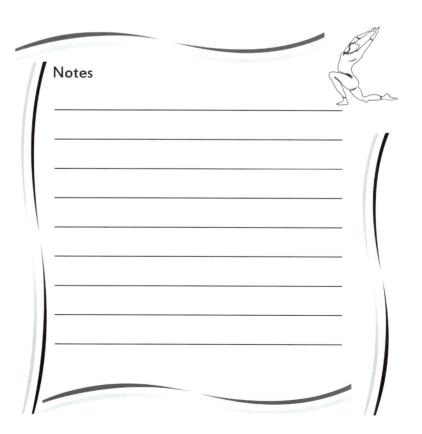

Notes

_____

_____

_____

_____

_____

_____

_____

_____

_____

I want to play with the gods

I want to play with the gods

Buddha at my right hand

Dance in the fields with Jesus

Drawing circles in the sand

I want to ride on moonbeams

Sip wine with legends of old

Frolic in the waves with Elijah

Become a parable untold

I want to know of ancient days

Follow rainbows as a master

Stand on mountains with Krishna

Sail the universe, only faster

I want to walk with the gods

Singing with beautiful Mary

Lying in the fountains of stardust

At twilight with folk of Fairy

I want to gaze at light shadows

Sprinkle dewdrops with the sages

Watch an Epoch grow with Enoch

Countless moments on my pages

-Jaylee Balch-

C
H
O
I
C
E

Picture a jester walking along his path in life. He carries his staff with a little bundle on one end, enough for his journey, without having a great burden to bear. He has been invited to the Cosmic Wedding!

The fool reaches a part of his journey where he finds the path splits into three different roads. As he looks at the first road on his left it says "The Spiritual Road." There are a number of Fakirs lying on beds of nails who have been meditating under trees for twenty years. They have been fasting and abstaining from sex and many things in life, those following strict dogmas.

He says to himself, That looks like a hard spiritual road and I don't feel that is for me. (Often many get caught up in the dogmas and rules of the spiritual systems and become caught in karma.) Next he notices the next road in front of him saying, "The Hard Road." He sees knights in shining armour ready to do battle, to fight their way through life, full of ego, wanting to be perfect and prove to the world what they are capable of.

The fool looks at these guys and says, "I am not a fighter and I would not last in battle with them, so the hard road is not for me." The next road says, "The Royal Road." The fool says, "I am in trouble because there is nothing royal about me."

Just then, the fool, being in touch with nature, sees a little white dove. The bird of intuition. As he becomes engrossed with the bird, he accidentally steps into the Royal Road and a guardian appears.

The guardian asks, "Where doth thou go?" The fool says, "I am sorry, I didn't mean to step in your road. I have been invited to the Cosmic Wedding and I am trying to find my way." The guardian says, "You may proceed." The fool, enjoying the journey like a child, finding wonder in everything by giving value to nothing, comes across another guardian and this one asks, "Where are you going and why?"

The fool replies, "I am going to the Cosmic Wedding and I am going there because I have been invited." The guardian says, "You may proceed."

You see, if you know where you are going in life, you will observe that the world will step aside and make things possible for you. Eventually, the three roads meet and the fool sees that spiritual beings from the other paths are there too. The three roads merge into one and in the middle of the road is a set of scales. On one side of the scale is a feather and on the other side is the place where you need to place your heart.

If you are weighed down from your experiences and still holding on to them, your heart will be too heavy and you will not be allowed to enter the wedding of the Cosmic Marriage. The people from the first road place their hearts on the scales, and ONLY those who have gone beyond the dogmas, rituals, and burdens find their hearts are light as a feather and they pass through. Then there are the knights with their now not-so-shiny armour, as they have been in battle, so proud of being a self-made person and the people they had to step on to make it to the top. They are battle-worn and tired and weighed down with their experiences, so when they hop on the scale, it dips down and their hearts are too heavy and they do not pass. It is then their lot to reincarnate again. The fool experienced life, although he held on to nothing and enjoyed life. The fool hops on the scale and is allowed to enter.

Applying this to your life is offering you an opportunity to step onto the Royal Road.

Practical exercises addressing CHOICE:

Exercise 1: Write down and reflect upon which road you have been on in which areas and at what stages in your life.

Exercise 2: Begin to make new choices! Each time you choose, your choice is an evaluation of yourself. You can do it the hard, self-sacrificing way, you can fight for everything you want, or you can choose to have fun, be mindful, take nothing too seriously (especially yourself), and let go of attachments!

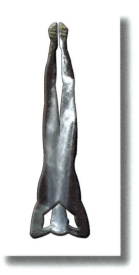

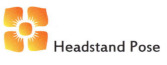

Headstand Pose

Salamba Sirasana

An inversion posture brings heaven back to earth by bringing the crown centre to the ground. This is the whole spiritual path to create the qualities of where you are going after this life, while you are in this life. This is what is meant by the statement "the steps of getting to where you want to be are the qualities of being there," by Lazaris. In other words, you need to draw the energy of the future into your present, and then you are on the right path.

Imagine your future and allow those qualities to lead you towards your future. Remember: You cannot create something that you don't know without having some sort of feelings about it. Simply sit and imagine, feel the success and what it feels like, and see yourself in that future. In this way, you have already begun to draw upon it. We always declare that what you want is up to you but how you get it is not. So dream your dream and allow the universe to present ways for you to walk towards your dream and take action when those opportunities arise. Each step is one closer to your dream.

BRING HEAVEN BACK TO EARTH...

It also includes:

- tapping the magic in the mundane
- seeing the beauty in all things and being willing to learn from all experiences no matter what they are
- seeing the extraordinary in the ordinary, where you make everything an opportunity to grow and learn and to create a result that is better than if the situation never happened.

MAKE THE PROPER ARRANGEMENTS, BEFORE YOU ARRIVE AT YOUR FUTURE...

This posture relates to creating a shift in perception, like the hanged man in the tarot, and being able to change your point of view to eventually having many viewing points. One must be careful to not indulge in the new perceptions, as they can trap you from continuously growing and evolving. People learn something new and then indulge in it and embellish it to make themselves seem as if they have evolved more than they really have. Celebrate what you have learnt and then move on. This posture allows more energy to awaken the psychic centres in the brain. This eventually awakens your subtle senses where you can sense and explore the subtle energies beyond the physical level of consciousness.

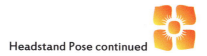

HEALING CONSIDERATIONS:

SHIFT YOUR CONSCIOUSNESS

BRING THE SPIRITUAL INTO THE PHYSICAL

CHANGE YOUR POINT OF VIEW—HAVE A 360-DEGREE VIEWING POINT

BRING THE MAGIC INTO THE MUNDANE—ENJOY EVERY MOMENT

BE EXCEPTIONAL, NOT THE EXCEPTION

WHAT SAVES A MAN IS TO TAKE A STEP. THEN ANOTHER STEP. IT IS ALWAYS THE SAME STEP, BUT YOU HAVE TO TAKE IT.
- ANTOINE DE SAINT-EXUPERY -

FIND THE MAGIC IN THE MUNDANE...

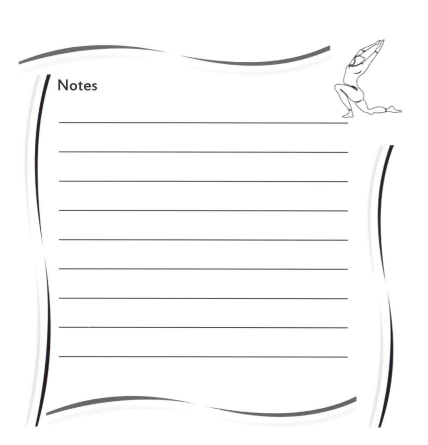

Notes

_____

_____

_____

_____

_____

_____

_____

_____

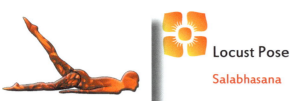

Locust Pose

Salabhasana

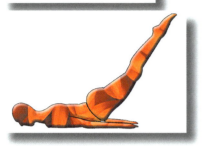

When you are kicking up the single leg lift (left or right side), you are working much deeper into the pelvic and buttock area. This movement can trigger shame. As explained in another posture, once again, many people are brought up by shame-based parents. They were either superhuman (highly accomplished, educated, and/ or wealthy) or they were subhuman (alcoholic, abusive, and in poverty). With the superhuman parents, they either expected you to be perfect or told you that you would never be as good as they were.

Always pushing, forcing, encouraging, and seldom actually celebrating your successes and achievements. Even if you scored high marks or received the gold medal, you were congratulated but told to do better next time. The actual achievement was never fully explored.

IF AT FIRST YOU DO SUCCEED, TRY NOT TO LOOK SO ASTONISHED...

The subhuman parents often abused you either mentally, physically, sexually, or emotionally and made you feel flawed and not good enough. This often leads to feelings of inadequacy and thinking you have done something wrong. You are here to express all aspects of yourself constructively and impeccably. This posture helps you release fear around expression. You need to express your power, and this is done by taking responsibility, which is being able to choose the optimum response and feeling secure and stable.

LOOK AT YOUR SUCCESSES, MEDIATE ON THEM, ABSORB THEM AND CELEBRATE THEM.

In the double leg lift, self-sabotage manifests—and relates to—not celebrating your successes. When you make a mistake, what do you do? You try to learn from it, take it apart, analyse it, and go into the details—don't you? When you have a success, do you do the same thing? NO! You smile and move on. Learn from your successes. What you learn from your mistakes is what NOT to do in life, and then you create a mediocre life, because you are not learning about success. Look at your successes, mediate on them, absorb them, and celebrate them.

Self-sabotage is also flirting with the negative ego: You race too fast in the car and think you will get away with it. You do dangerous things, like shooting up heroin, and you believe you are invincible and superhuman. Sooner or later, you come crashing down from your perception.

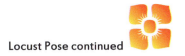

Healing considerations:

Release shame

Release self-sabotage

Be motivated out of caring and not concern

Balance your emotional centre

Feel and let go

Create realistic aspirations and dreams

Encourage concentration and perseverance

Forgive your parents; they tried their best

Forgive yourself; you tried your best

Yoga has a sly, clever way of short-circuiting the mental patterns that cause anxiety.

~Baxter Bell -

Notes

_____

_____

_____

_____

_____

_____

_____

_____

_____

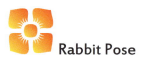

Rabbit Pose

Sasangasana

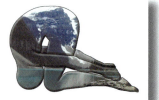

Rabbit Pose is the opposite of Camel Pose—it has a very strong front side compression and it is an inversion posture, so it activates all seven chakras. It is probably the main inversion posture, because the top of your head touches the ground. Your Crown Centre (on the top of your head) relates to your Unlimited Potential, so you are bringing your Unlimited Potential into physical manifestation to stretch beyond what you are capable of. Bringing heaven back to earth! Your earth can be heaven or it can be hell; it is your perception of the beliefs or choices that govern this. With this front side compression, it is another posture that is good for releasing martyrhood, as it works deeply into the pancreas area.

A RABBIT BRINGS HEAVEN BACK TO EARTH...

The whole back area relates to that which you have buried and hidden behind you all your life. In this posture you actually elongate your spine (this posture can open up the spine up to 350 millimetres), opening up the spaces and allowing that which has been suppressed and repressed to come to the surface to be released. The shadow is made up of all the aspects of yourself and your life that you deny and defend yourself against and all the aspects that you pretend don't exist. All the ugly stuff of your life is here. Your shadow is also made up of all the power and talents that you pretend you don't have and all your gifts that you have to use and offer yourself and your world.

YOUR SHADOW HOLDS YOUR DARK AND LIGHT SIDE...

You were taught to be afraid to go into your shadow because that is where the real truth lies. This is where your internal voice doesn't want you to go, because you then have the possibility to transcend the dark side and tap into your talents and become an amazing expression of what life can be. You have to be very strong in abdominal area to break through facades, the image you hide behind. The alter ego will lie to you and tell you, 'you are the worst' or 'you are the greatest'. The shadow is part of your subconscious mind that tells you the truth—it does not lie to you. Most people don't deal with their darkness and therefore rob themselves of their light. When you have exaggerated emotions regarding a situation, it is a big indicator that you have triggered the dark side of your shadow. Your response is over the top regarding the situation. For example, you leave your shoes in the wrong place and once again and your partner/parent screams and threatens you. Their anger and rage has been suppressed over years and has been denied and placed in the shadow. Now it is being expressed in the moment over the shoes, but there is far too much emotion and intensity for the situation. The dark side of your shadow pushes you into situations, and the light side of your shadow pulls you into them.

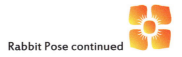

HEALING CONSIDERATIONS:

ALLOW YOUR SHADOW TO SURFACE

EXPRESS DEEP DESIRES AND LET GO OF PROJECTIONS

CLEAR EMOTIONAL ADDICTIONS

LET GO OF USING SMOKE SCREENS TO HIDE BEHIND

RELEASE YOUR SHADOW AND FEAR AROUND KNOWING THYSELF

WE ALL HAVE TO TASTE DIRT AT SOME POINT, BUT WHEN WE STAND, WE TASTE THE SUN. THERE IS A BALANCE IN EVERYTHING.

- JAYLEE B -

Notes

_____

_____

_____

_____

_____

_____

_____

_____

L
O
V
E

Paul came up with a wonderful concept: "Love is the force that takes us out of the delusion of separation." We are taught and spend our lives believing that we have to give in order to get. We are drummed with concepts of not being selfish and giving more, yet we are never taught to love ourselves.

If you are born with a cup of love and from the first moment you can remember you pass this cup around to everyone you come across, by the time the cup returns to you, what happens? It is empty, and when your cup is empty, what do you instinctively do? You begin to demand or expect others to replenish you once again.

Instead, if we are taught to fill our own cup continuously, what happens? Our cups fill up and it begins to overflow. It is the overflow that reaches others and we never find ourselves empty. So, love must be felt and experienced first by ourselves, towards ourselves, for ourselves. Then, and only then, can we share it with others.

"Love is not enough unless it is interwoven with self-esteem, intimacy, and the caring that comes from both. Similarly, self-love is not enough. You need to interweave with self-love loving someone more, which is one of the secrets of empowerment. This is the paradox. Do we mean loving someone more than yourself or do we mean loving someone who is more than you? Yes." —Lazaris

Most often, people confuse true love with the feelings of being in love. Being in love is simply a feel-good feeling based on a chemical reaction. Have you noticed how being in love diminishes after a few months or a year? It just isn't the same anymore. It is nice but it is not the high you once experienced.

Asked about love one day, we replied that there are three kinds of love. First, there is the love that comes from building memories. Everyone begins that way. Each moment is a living memory that accumulates. Most people think that stacking memories keeps them together! Memories are not glue when a relationship is flawed.

Secondly, some then accumulate reasons for being together. This can work as a glue, especially when the reasons are children. Many couples remain together although they are unsuitable or have fallen out of love or are very unhappy. Reasons such as monetary investments, contracts, children, the fear of being alone, the feeling that you would never find anyone else, being emotionally abused, and having no self-worth are just some of the reasons for staying with someone. There are very positive reasons for staying together, like the first time you danced, the moment you saw each other, the night you conceived the child, the holiday to Vegas, and many more, however, most relationships never go past this.

Thirdly, there is the unique relationship where memories and reasons are no longer the cohesive force. When a relationship hinges on the prior two, if one of them should cease to be of importance, the relationship can break—it is dependent on either memories or reasons.

With the third type of love, two people are together simply because they choose to be. They don't need a reason and they don't rely on memories—they simply are. If you take the memories away, nothing changes. If you take the reasons away, nothing changes.

It is a choice and they have made up their mind! This is the strongest relationship!

Practical exercises addressing LOVE:

Exercise: Take a good look at your various relationships. Where do they fit into the above three commitments?

Exercise: Are you giving to yourself? Are you loving you? If you don't, others won't! Are you loving you? If you don't, others won't!

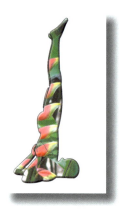

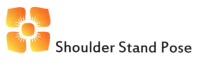

Shoulder Stand Pose

Salamba Sarvangasana

This posture does the same as Pranayama Breathing in releasing indecision by working on the neck. It also works on Expression through the Throat Centre. Having inverted the body, I would suggest this pose is about expressing the higher energies of wisdom, unlimited potentials, spiritual knowledge, and psychic awareness. Having inverted, you are like the Hanged Man (in the tarot deck), shifting perception from seeing one point of view to seeing many viewing points. In the same way you are able to see beyond your normal way of expressing yourself and opening up to many new ways of communicating and expressing. It also helps you to let go of the past and see life from a higher perception and awaken the subtle senses.

DON'T BE INDECISIVE - MAKE YOUR MIND UP AND TAKE ACTION...

When we let go of how we have seen the past, we actually change the past's influence upon us. We have actively chosen to look at the past, present, and the future in a new way. Our perception determines the influences we allow to impact us. Be willing to own and express the subtle things you pick up in life and not discount that you do have subtle abilities. You have heard that you can cut the air with a knife. Well, this relates to your subtle senses, or people having the same thought at the same time and thinking of someone just before they ring. All this relates to your subtle senses and they are natural.

Your future can impact and influence you greater than your past can, if you allow it to. That is why it is crucial that you have a dream. Your dream of your future will come back in time to begin changing you, so that you will be capable of manifesting your dream. For example, if you dream of owning a new sports car but have never taken your driver's license, your future, where you own the car, will impact upon you to go for your license so that you can manifest the car of your dreams AND enjoy it. All magicians know that the future is far more powerful to work with if they need to change their lives.

The psychic senses relate to subtle feedback mechanisms within us and they pick up vibrations of a subtle level that are incoming. Then, depending to what extent you are consciously awake, you can decipher and interpret them to gain a greater insight and have an edge in life. These abilities don't make you spiritual and they don't relate to the spiritual world; they are useful in the everyday world and everybody has the potential if utilised. The

128 more you encourage yourself, the more your mind and body will respond.

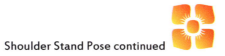

HEALING CONSIDERATIONS:

FORGET WHAT YOU
HAVE BEEN,
REMEMBER, INSTEAD
WHO YOU ARE
- JAYLEE B -

RELEASE THE INDECISION IN YOUR LIFE

LEARN TO EXPRESS THE WISDOM YOU HAVE ACCESS TO

LET GO OF THE PAST

BE OPEN TO PSYCHIC ABILITIES

ALLOW YOUR FUTURE TO CHANGE YOU

Notes

_____

_____

_____

_____

_____

_____

_____

_____

_____

_____

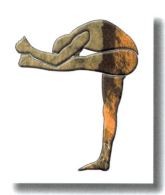

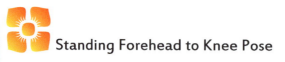

Standing Forehead to Knee Pose

Dandayamana Janushirasana

In life we tend to take ourselves far too seriously which the result is we become self important and look for external validation almost constantly. We also take our partners and family far too seriously, often allowing them to steal your peace in life. When we give our power away to others, we then need and often become dependent on them for validation.

YOU ARE TAKING LIFE TOO SERIOUSLY...

The more important we make people in our lives the more potential we have of giving power away to them and allow them to influence and control us through their actions and comments. We need to focus on being clear and letting go of the past emotional experiences and create a balance within ourselves. It has been said that this universe is a free will universe so we don't have the right to impose our beliefs and attitudes upon others. Most often, this is based upon judgment and maintains a separation. Remember what the bible says, "judge not least thy be judged".

Look at how you respond when you are with men and women and note the difference if any and why it is so. We need to be at home and be natural dealing with male and female energies within and without. You also need to be willing to trust and believe in yourself and live life to the full. Learn to focus and concentrate on yourself and let others be. There is an old Sufi story which goes something like this; there is a master and his pupil. The pupil goes to his master and says master how do we get rid of my undesirable friends, the master replies simply lead a desirable life and your undesirable friends will drop out of your life. We have been conditioned to show our gratitude by saying thank you, we would suggest that to really show gratitude for something you need to make the most of it. In other words if we look at life being a gift from the cosmic we then need to live life to the full to demonstrate our gratitude.

DON'T HOLD BACK AND BE A SPECTATOR!

Don't hold back and be a spectator, participate in the best game of all life, and play it as best you can. Now let's look at co dependencies in relationships. It manifests that you allow yourself to be controlled by the behaviour of your partner and vice versa. So you try to control their behaviour before it controls you and you end up dominating and manipulating each other. When your dependency becomes destructive then you have a co-dependency.

There are four criteria to co-dependency and the first is that it must involve a dependency that demands adherence to oppressive rules that limit or eliminate the open expression of thought and feeling or communication. We cannot talk about why we don't have sex, you must mow the lawn, this is how long you can talk on the phone etc. etc. The second criterion is that it is a dependency that diminishes your capacity to initiate or participate in loving relationships. It means that it diminishes your capacity to receive love. we cannot receive love from this person. They are drunk, abusive, violent, self destructive etc. Also there is no way we can give. we can't give them security, pleasure, a sense of vulnerability, trust or intimacy.

Why do you want to go out? You can't have friends. That is a co dependant relationship. The third criteria is that it is a co-dependency when the behaviour of the other person seems to control your life and when you become obsessed in controlling their controlling behaviours in order to be free. we must get them to stop drinking before we can be happy, we must get them to get a decent job and then we can sleep at night, we must get them to grow and then we can be spiritual etc. etc. My freedom, happiness and independence has nothing with me, it has everything to do with fixing and controlling them and getting them to change.

And the fourth criterion is that it is a dependency that exaggerates the need to control thus producing the insatiable need for outside validation. It is such a crippling dependency that you become woefully self neglectful. You don't sleep or eat etc. etc. and becomes destructive and masochistic.

Too serious = you make something too real and therefore when you program it to change it doesn't work because the more it becomes fixed in an illusionary world and it can't work.

> "THERE IS NO SUCH THING AS A PROBLEM WITHOUT A GIFT FOR YOU IN ITS HANDS. WE SEEK OUT PROBLEMS BECAUSE WE NEED THEIR GIFTS."
> ~ RICHARD BACH -

HEALING CONSIDERATIONS:

EXPRESS AND RELEASE RESENTMENT AND ANGER TOWARDS PAST RELATIONSHIPS

NEUTRALISE YOUR CO-DEPENDENCIES

FORGIVE YOUR JUDGMENT TOWARDS OTHERS

STRENGTHEN YOUR RELATIONSHIP WITH YOURSELF

BALANCE THE MALE AND FEMALE ENERGIES

Standing Separate Leg Stretching Pose

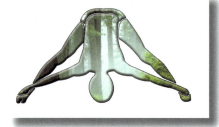

Dandayamana Bibhaktapada Paschimatthanasana

This posture is a front side compression and an inversion posture that is working all seven chakras. As discussed in other postures, you are working the pancreas through the front side compression, which relates to martyrhood. Martyrhood is about giving until it hurts and putting yourself second.

DON'T GIVE UNTIL IT HURTS...

When you give to the extent that you are taken advantage of, you end up feeling not appreciated and martyring yourself. Often people who need to do this are in need of external validation and so they give in to the hope that everyone will appreciate them and give them the validation they need to feel good enough. When a person is caught up in martyr they are master manipulators because they will manipulate through feeling sorry for themselves and thus control others to help them. When you control others you are breaking a law of the universe that states that you are not allowed to interfere with someone's free will. If you do, you then give permission for your free will to be interfered with, so reap as you sow.

Because it is an inversion posture, you are changing thought patterns and releasing resentment, through the connection of your forehead to your knee—resentment because of emotional scars from the past.

RELEASE THE EMOTIONAL SCARS OF THE PAST

In the past, you emotionally opened up to someone, became vulnerable, and you were hurt and wounded. It takes a while for the wound to heal, but it eventually does; however, you don't allow yourself to let go of the memory and it forms an energetic scar. The scar is a reminder of that past hurt and it does not allow you to let go.

Love creates an opportunity for you to show love and do the loving. Gaining the benefit of love comes more from loving than from getting love. Love is freedom—it is not the expectation of roles and rules and boundaries. Love is not bondage. A relationship is the interaction between two people. Your partner is not the relationship.

Release the emotional scars towards the people in your past—the right-hand side is resentment towards males in your past who have wounded you, and on the left- hand side, you release resentment towards females in your past who have wounded you.

We tend to allow our minds to indulge in old painful experiences and replay them over

and over. By doing so we end up creating a neuro-net that filters our perception of reality and only draws those scenarios repeatedly back to ourselves. We are also reenergising and reinforcing those experiences, so they have a bigger influence over us in our present lives. We need to let go and die to those past experiences, including the beautiful ones, as they can also hold us back through reminiscing. We then only create what we have already experienced in our past and not something new and more. When these thoughts manifest in your mind say "thank you but no thank you," let them go, and replace them with a new thought of what you do want. This is assuming you know what you want.

Let go of the emotional scars of the past. To do this you need to forgive yourself and those you have allowed to trespass against you. You see, the important aspect is to own that you have allowed people to trespass against you, and as you accept this, you are empowered to change the impact.

Many people end up punishing themselves over a past relationship as a way to punish those people that they allowed to hurt them. By holding on to the pain, you are stopping yourself from moving on, even though those who were involved moved on long ago. If you are blaming others, then you cannot change the impact, because through blame you have become powerless and are believing that you want the person responsible to come and fix you and your situation.

> IRRIGATORS DIRECT THE WATER, ARCHERS FASHION THE SHAFT, CARPENTERS CARVE THE WOOD, THE WISE CONTROL THEMSELVES.
> - SANSKRIT -

> LET GO OF TAKING YOURSELF TOO SERIOUSLY...

HEALING CONSIDERATIONS:

RELEASE THE RESENTMENTS OF THE PAST

RELEASE THE SCARS CAUSED BY HURT

EMERGE FROM YOUR COCOON AS A TRANSFORMED PERSON

LET GO OF FORCING YOURSELF TO BE RID OF THE PAST

DEAL WITH THOSE NEGATIVE EMOTIONS

FORGIVE THOSE WHO HAVE ERRED AGAINST YOU

LEARN THAT ONLY YOU CAN CHANGE YOUR PAST DON'T WAIT FOR SOMEONE ELSE TO FIX YOU

CHANGE

Change creates challenges, which prompts you to reassess where you are at and where you want to go in your life. Change is an opportunity that offers you new possibilities in life. Change challenges you to make new decisions and take responsibility in your lives. Change is a mystery because it happens instantaneously, and all you can do is experience the effect and the influence of the change. Buddha said, "The only thing that doesn't change is change is continuous." You tend to feel inertia and a resistance to change because it pulls us out of your comfort zone and you feel threatened and destabilized. This can plunge you into the dark side chaos, in which you are overwhelmed and confronted with the many options that change brings.

Change is an energy that you cannot see all you can do is allow the effect of change to take place because it happens instantly within you and the effects unfold outside of you if you allow them. Our whole world is changing rapidly. With the changes you enter into chaos. You either enter the light side of chaos, which relates to freedom with its many choices or the dark side of chaos with its confusion, doubt, and depression and you are forced to either make a choice to change or shut down emotionally.

You cannot control change, you can only have control of yourself as the effects of change unfold around you, and then you can respond to the changes. Change begins with your dreams of a better future, and the energy is projected on to your future and then comes back into your present to make the changes necessary for you to reach that desired goal/dream. The change needs to take place within your subconscious mind, as that part of your mind is running your life and it is much more powerful than your conscious mind. You need to stop worrying about the changes and allow them to unfold. We tend to get in our own way of harnessing the effects of the changes we have set in motion through looking for the effects and trying to make them happen, which never works.

The two energies that are a big part of change are choice and image. Change comes from choice and choice comes from image; they work together. To transcend the way you see yourself is what produces the change. If you make choices and create new images and hold them in your mind's eye, your subconscious mind will receive them and change will occur. It is important to embrace change; otherwise you will be left behind living an image in an old time zone, which ends up being lost.

A friend in Sydney found that carrot juice was good for you, so he was having a few gallons a day. He lost one kidney and he almost lost the second one as well. Everything in moderation is the best approach. This program is designed upon principals based on ancient knowledge and is being updated regularly to accommodate our ever-changing, modern lifestyle.

Question: Would you like to change the way you respond to change?

Practical exercises addressing LOVE:

Exercise 1: Write down your thoughts for ten minutes per day for twenty-eight days, listening to the little voice that is in your mind.

Exercise 2: Write down your five main fears and resistances to change.

Exercise 3: Write down five main exciting times when you embraced change.

Exercise 4: Write down what you would like to change in your life now.

Exercise 5: Practice an emotional relaxation meditation daily (to be done for a minimum of ten minutes and a maximum of thirty minutes).

Exercise 6: exercise 5 is to be done for a minimum of ten minutes and a maximum of 30 minutes. We found from the years of experimenting that 10 minutes minimum and a maximum of half an hour practicing the mind exercise is optimum. After that it becomes counter productive. You need to be practical and sensible with your practices.

LEAVES ARE LIGHT, AND USELESS, AND IDLE,
AND WAVERING, AND CHANGEABLE; THEY EVEN DANCE;
AND YET GOD IN HIS WISDOM HAS MADE THEM
A PART OF OAKS.
AND IN SO DOING HE HAS GIVEN US A LESSON,
NOT TO DENY THE STOUT-HEARTEDNESS WITHIN
BECAUSE WE SEE THE LIGHTSOMENESS WITHOUT.
~AUGUSTUS WILLIAM HARE AND
JULIUS CHARLES HARE, 1827 -

GEYSER - YELLLOWSTONE NATIONAL PARK

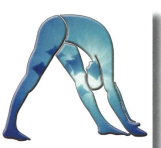

Standing Separate Leg Head to Knee Pose

Dandayamana Bibhaktapada Janushirasana

We tend to allow our mind to indulge in old painful experiences and replay them over and over. By doing so, we end up creating a neurone that filters our perception of reality, and only draws those scenarios to ourselves. We are also re – energising and reinforcing those experiences so they have a bigger influence over us in our present life. We need to let go and die to those past experiences including the beautiful ones as they can also hold us back through reminiscing to only what we experienced in our past hence recreating our past and not something new and more.

LET GO OF THE EMOTIONAL SCARS OF THE PAST...

When these thoughts manifest in your mind say thank you but no thankyou and let them go and replace them with a new thought of what you want. This is assuming you know what you want. Let go of the emotional scars of the past and to do this you need to forgive yourself and those you have allowed to trespass against you. See the important aspect is to own that you have allowed people to trespass against you and as you accept this then you are empowered to change the impact. Many people end up punishing themselves over a past relationship as a way to punish those people that they allowed to hurt them. By holding onto the pain, stopping them from moving on even though those who were involved have moved on long ago.

BECOME RESPONSIBLE FOR YOUR OWN HEALING JOURNEY...

If you are blaming others then you cannot change the impact because through blame you become disempowered and are saying that you want the person responsible to come and fix you and your situation. When you give to the extent that you are taken advantage of you end up feeling not appreciated and martyring yourself.

DANCE LIKE NO ONE IS LOOKING, LOVE LIKE YOU HAVE NEVER BEEN HURT...

Often people who need to do this are in need of external validation and so they give in the hope that everyone will appreciate them and give them the validation they need to feel good enough. When a person is caught up in martyr they are master manipulators because they will manipulate through feeling sorry for themselves and thus control others to help them. When you control others you are breaking a law of the universe which states you are not allowed to interfere with someone's free will. If you do you then give permission for your free will to be interfered with, reap as you sow.

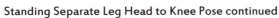

HEALING CONSIDERATIONS:

LET GO OF OLD THOUGHT PATTERNS REGARDING PAST RELATIONSHIPS,

RELEASING THE EMOTIONAL SCARS FROM PAST RELATIONSHIPS,

LET GO OF CONTROLLING RELATIONSHIPS,

RELEASE MENTAL BLOCKS,

LET GO OF TAKING YOUR THOUGHTS TOO SERIOUSLY.

ENHANCE YOUR OUTWARD EXPRESSION OR INWARD ACCEPTANCE

THE FUTURE LIES BEFORE YOU, LIKE PATHS OF PURE WHITE SNOW. BE CAREFUL HOW YOU TREAD IT, FOR EVERY STEP WILL SHOW.
~AUTHOR UNKNOWN -

Notes

_____

_____

_____

_____

_____

_____

_____

_____

_____

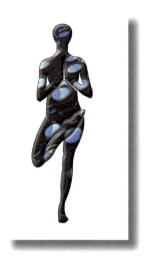

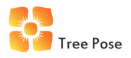

Tree Pose

Tadasana

Opening the pelvic region and bringing the ankle up onto the groin area releases the need to flirt sexually. We have been brought up with the in-built program to flirt with others of the opposite sex to ensure there will be more humans and our species will survive. This is a natural on an animal level for procreation to take place. When we allow our negative ego to get a hold of this and we are very focused on our external image and validation, we package ourselves in a way to sexually flirt and get attention and energy from others.

RELEASE THE NEED TO FLIRT OUTRAGEOUSLY...

The term "control drama" is mentioned in the book The Celestine Prophecy, and this is what is manifesting through flirting. You are behaving in a way to create an impact to get attention and energy. Often what takes place is that you end up receiving people's sexual energies projected on to you, which may not be the best for you in the long run, depending upon whether the person's intentions are pure or not.

Many men and women need to flirt to get the attention of others to feel that they are good enough. This usually happens because of feeling insecure and having low self-esteem and a poor relationship with oneself. This feeds their negative ego's need for external validation and this puts you at the mercy of those with whom you need attention from. This happens when you don't own your own power and presence.

IT IS NATURAL TO HAVE FANTASIES, HOWEVER...

This posture can help to break through your sexual programming and the fear of being sexually betrayed, so you can express yourself freely and fully. Society's programming around sex, especially through various religious and spiritual practices, have restricted, judged, and controlled the exploration and celebration of sexuality. We have suppressed and repressed our sexuality to such a degree that unfortunately many have sexually-based issues. It is a natural thing to have dreams and fantasies; however, it is a lack of integrity to cultivate thoughts about others while you are cultivating a relationship with a partner, as this is a type of betrayal.

Another form of sexual betrayal is working to such a degree that you are exhausted and you lack motivation to connect sexually with your partner. Your message is that your job is taking precedence over your sexual and intimate life. Sexual energy is a beautiful energy to be harnessed and celebrated; it relates to the primal energy of creation, which is to be used to create on all levels.

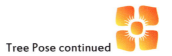

HEALING CONSIDERATIONS:

RELEASE FEAR OF BETRAYAL

RELEASE THE NEED FOR SEXUAL FLIRTING

FIND SECURITY IN SEXUAL EXPRESSION

FREE UP YOUR SELF-EXPRESSION AND PAST EMOTIONAL

RELATIONSHIP EXPERIENCES

"DIFFICULT TIMES HAVE HELPED ME TO UNDERSTAND BETTER THAN BEFORE, HOW INFINITELY RICH AND BEAUTIFUL LIFE IS IN EVERY WAY, AND THAT SO MANY THINGS THAT ONE GOES WORRYING ABOUT ARE OF NO IMPORTANCE WHATSOEVER."

~ ISAK DINESEN -

Notes

_____

_____

_____

_____

_____

_____

_____

_____

_____

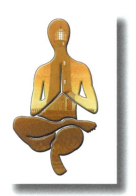

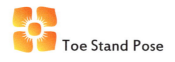

Toe Stand Pose
Padangustasana

n this posture, you are working the ankles and deeply into the pelvic region and your foot is coming up on to the groin area, activating the Sacral Centre. Strangely, many have an innate fear of being of being sexually rejected and this has a different impact upon men than women. It is important to let go of the sexual expectations of performance and be totally present. Sexuality is an expression of your soul through the sharing of your physical, emotional, mental, and spiritual bodies with another. Let go of the judgements towards yourself sexually and accept your sexual identity. Even when you are in a relationship, you have the right to say no and so does your partner, and it is not always a reflection of how unattractive or unworthy you are. It is best to connect with your partner when you are BOTH in the right space.

WHO SUFFERS FROM SEXUAL REJECTION?

Which gender do you think feels the pangs of sexual rejection more? Ponder this!

The easiest way for someone to create is to bring the God and the Goddess together, forming a union. What does it mean to be a man? What does it mean to be a woman?

Have you ever sat and actually thought about it? We have definite measurements of what a woman is: 26-32-26measurements, for instance, or as a man, he has a great car and good looks. So often, we fall into the current age's ideals about what a woman or man is that we don't even stop to think about how we feel. Is a woman about sex, make-up, kids, or shoes? Is a man about biceps, car, salary, or beer? Surely, we are much more. We are not our bodies. Our bodies are simply the vehicles that carry our souls around. We are very much about our consciousness or our spiritualness. This makes the difference in how we suffer from or process information, learn lessons, and what we attract into our lives. Give this thought and change your life.

HEALING CONSIDERATIONS:

CREATE BALANCE AND FOCUS IN YOUR BODY AND MIND

STRENGTHEN YOUR SEXUAL IDENTITY AND GENDER

SHARE YOUR EMOTIONAL AND SPIRITUAL SIDES

SURRENDER TO THIS POSTURE AND FOCUS ON CHANGE

RELEASE JUDGEMENTS ABOUT WHO YOU THINK YOU ARE

Ever wondered who held the pen

Ever wonder who held the pen

When you first took your breath

Who scribbled yours tears and falls down stairs

Or who penned your joys and birthday gifts

And potty trained you under duress of ink

With screams and mistakes in the mix

Who chose the boy in the denim shirt

With the shy smile and lanky swagger

To be your first love and to break your heart

For you to be determined to achieve

Who grew your hair with strokes of lead

Pencilled in just in case you needed change

And scratched in honesty, temperance and joy

To greet you each day you awoke from off the page

Who gave your hand in marriage on your twenty first

When your life was only beginning

Ever wonder who held the pen

When your baby took its first breath

Who coloured the page with your mothering charm

And tears of joy at your child's first step

When you sang softly in the nursery or needed a break

Who gave you a mirror to appreciate your wrinkles

Or Pencilled in the grey streaks in mid winter

Just before spring when you coloured it again

Who jotted the hope of a loving and fruitful life

When you signed your will over to a baldy man

Because you had no memories or wit

Who scribed you into a home for the dying

When you felt on top of the world all the time

Ever wonder who held the pen

When you laid down this body and took your first breath

-Jaylee Balch

MAGNETISM

Magnetism relates to charisma, presence, and the ability to influence and attract what you want in life. When using magnetism, you create a genuine win/win situation, due to the principle of induction.

To build your personal magnetism, you need to stretch the neck and keep the spine straight, raising your chest a bit to allow the spinal life force energy to flow more effectively. Imagine you are trying to touch the ceiling with the top of your head. Learn to adopt this position in everything you do and also learn to walk without jarring the brain stem. When you are in your car, move your mirror so that you sit with your head reaching towards the roof, as this also trains you to maintain a straight, but not ridged, spine.

To build magnetism, you need to make an effort to stop short of feeling full when you eat, because overeating diminishes your personal magnetism. If you take a magnet and rub it on a nail, thus magnetising the nail, your magnet will not be less of a magnet than it was before. It could magnetise a million nails and still maintain its magnetic properties. You can lose personal magnetism through superficial thoughts. Many articles can be considered mental desserts, but they lack the power to stretch your mind and develop the ability to think laterally, diagonally, and vertically. Fidgeting drains personal magnetism, so practicing stillness of mind and body develops it.

Magnetism has to do with the personal space within you. The sense of feeling you have within you radiates around you. As you reflect upon the space within, you ponder upon the relationships you have with the people closest in your life. How these people respond towards you is a reflection of the space you are in when you deal with them. Look at the qualities they possess and reflect upon these as aspects of yourself or aspects you need to cultivate within you. Many people compete and compare themselves with others. What this does is rob you of your individuality and uniqueness. If you respect and love yourself, you will demonstrate this towards others naturally. According to the personal space within you, you will attract or be drawn to specific people and situations in life.

You need to focus upon the good within everyone and offer them your best always. As you live this way of life, you will change the personal space within you and create an impeccable impact wherever you go in life. Opportunities will just manifest out of the blue, like miracles. By operating this way, it will eventually become an automatic way of life where miracles happen every day.

An old saying we follow: What you see outside of yourself is what you grow within.

One evening, an old Cherokee told his grandson about a battle that goes on inside people. He said, "My son, the battle is between two 'wolves' inside all of us. One is evil. It is anger, envy, jealousy, sorrow, regret, greed, arrogance, self-pity, guilt, resentment, inferiority, lies, faults, pride, superiority, and ego. The other is good. It is joy, peace, love, hope, serenity, humility, kindness, benevolence, empathy, generosity, truth, compassion, and faith."

The grandson contemplated for about a minute and then asked his grandfather, "Which wolf wins?"

The old Cherokee simply replied, "The one you feed."

Practical exercises addressing MAGNETISM:

Exercise 1: Evaluate and write down what percentage of the time you dwell on negative outcomes.

Exercise 2: Become conscious of focusing on constructive thoughts from now on.

Exercise 3: What is the quality of space within you?

Exercise 4: Be honest! Do friends long to be with you or make excuses to avoid you?

IT NEEDS AN EXTRAORDINARILY ASTUTE MIND,
AN EXTRAORDINARILY PLIABLE HEART, TO BE AWARE OF AND TO FOL-
LOW WHAT IS; BECAUSE WHAT IS, IS CONSTANTLY MOVING, CONSTANTLY
UNDERGOING TRANSFORMATION, AND IF THE MIND IS TETHERED TO
BELIEF,
TO KNOWLEDGE, IT CEASES TO PURSUE, IT CEASES TO FOLLOW THE
SWIFT MOVEMENT OF WHAT IS.
- KRISHNAMURTI -

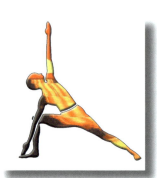

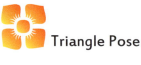

Triangle Pose

Trikanasana

This is Triangle Pose—top of floor series (in Hot Yoga). It is connecting all the heart energies—working the elbows, knees, and hips and opening the chest. This posture changes the blood chemistry by working deeply through the torso and hips. It has a lot to do with releasing emotional addictions. We are constantly re-creating emotional patterns, which reoccur over and over, like emotional dramas.

BIGGEST HEART OPENING POSTURE...

Most people in a relationship have an addiction to a feel-good -feeling—"You make me feel happy, so I am going to hang out with you. I am going to call it love, and when you stop creating that feel-good feeling for me, I am going to fall out of love with you very quickly. When you are cooking for me, earning money for me, and taking care of me, I will love you. If you stop, I will no longer love you."

WHY ARE WOMEN SEEN AS SEX OBJECTS...? MEN ARE SEEN AS SUCCESS OBJECTS... WHY?

Are you hard on yourself? Triangle helps to release stubbornness—stubbornness towards yourself, so forgive yourself and appreciate yourself. You are too busy driving yourself into the ground. Release your masochistic tendencies, very hard towards yourself. Let go of the fear of being emotionally vulnerable! Open that chest and front side! It is a strength to be vulnerable, not a weakness. Give yourself love and forgiveness and change your habits by doing things differently. Have a different attitude towards a posture each time you walk into the room. The postures you tend to avoid are the postures you need the most. There is a resistance!

This posture releases stubborn anger aimed towards you from yourself. You need to balance your self-image through looking at how you see yourself and how the world sees you. Remember that the way the world sees you is their interpretation of who you were in that moment and not who you really are in the big scheme of things. This posture helps you to release the fear around being loving and receiving love. Do you feel worthy to receive someone's love? Let go of the restrictions around love and relationships.

DO THINGS DIFFERENTLY...

Let go of the resistances, judgements, and fears relating to old past relationships. Release the fear around your love changing and evolving. Many try to keep the love they have static because they fear losing the love. What happens is you fear losing the focal point of your love, and the more you love the more you potentially have to lose, according to Lazaris. This can hold you back from loving like you have never been hurt before, loving fully and freely.

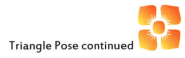

To what extent do you love yourself? How do you demonstrate this self-love in life? Let go of beating yourself up and being angry at yourself and it is time to finally accept yourself and allow yourself to be fully loved. While you are hard and angry at yourself you will not allow the love from others to reach you. Be willing to receive the love others have for you and be willing to show your love more for those who care. Look at how you treat yourself and whether you are your own best friend or worst enemy. Learn to forgive, accept, support, and love yourself.

Don't give up on yourself. Release the shield that you have placed around your heart to protect yourself because this is holding you back from knowing yourself. It is time to feel your emotions, express them, and find a balance. Everyone has the same spiritual worth; it is only how you choose to see it that makes you feel you are worthless. Where does this voice come from? The altered or negative ego.

IF YOU START JUDGING PEOPLE, YOU WILL BE HAVING NO TIME TO LOVE THEM
— MOTHER TERESA -

RELEASE THE SHIELD AROUND YOUR HEART…

HEALING CONSIDERATIONS:

RELEASE THE RESENTMENT TOWARDS NOT RECEIVING ENOUGH LOVE IN RELATIONSHIPS

HELPS TO REGULATE HORMONE LEVELS TO CLEAR EMOTIONAL ADDICTIONS

LEARN TO CARE MORE FOR FAMILY—REMEMBER BLOOD IS THICKER THAN WATER

EXPRESS AND RELEASE ANGER AND RESISTANCE AROUND SELF-LOVE AND VULNERABILITY

RELEASE MENTAL AND EMOTIONAL RIGIDITY AND INFLEXIBILITY

RELEASE THE FEAR AROUND LOVING

ENHANCE YOUR SELF-IMAGE AND SELF-LOVE

LET GO OF LOW SELF-ESTEEM AND SELF-WORTH

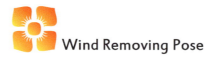

Wind Removing Pose

Pavanamuktasana

You are working the pelvic area, hips, and abdominal area. Your neck is flat, triggering the thyroid and activating the communication and expression centre.

Lifting the right leg is addressing how you communicate to your world. Compressing the intestines means you need to examine how you give and receive on an emotional level. When we function from a spiritual level, we do the right thing because it is the right thing to do, but when we get caught in the monkey mind, we do things for our own personal gain. Be impeccable in all your interactions. As you sow, so you shall reap. What goes around, comes around.

WHAT GOES AROUND, COMES AROUND...

Lifting the left leg is about emotional attachments to the past and those conflicts and challenges that you hold on to. Constipation is refusing to let go of the past; diarrhoea is trying to force yourself to let go of the past. When we are stressed, we tighten our sphincter muscle and this affects the bowel and colon and can cause haemorrhoids.

Both knees to chest, constricting your throat, and working the pelvic area develops a personal magnetic energetic space and that energy permeates your environment. You have a powerful impact and you have an impact even by your presence—there are no spectators in life, only participators. Take ownership for your impact and make it count.

Let go of the expectation of error and anxiety when you refuse to acknowledge that you have anger, hurt, self-pity, or fear. You expect to make a mistake; you expect to do it wrong. Release the idea of anticipating rejection or humiliation. Misplaced trust can hold you back from receiving abundance and love and comes when you have doubt.

This posture helps you let go of what is redundant in your life. Far too often the things we remember and hold on to don't serve us anymore, so we need to let them go. Some of these memories are unpleasant ones and we keep replaying them, and we need to ask ourselves why we constantly replay certain memories. Some of those redundant memories are pleasant ones, like replaying the good times that once were and wishing for them again. This means you will recreate the past and not actually grow and move into something new, which could actually be more than what you have experienced before.

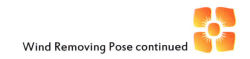

The important thing is to gain the value through processing your experiences and then let go of them so you create more room for the next experience to arrive.

NOTHING IS IMPOSSIBLE — THE WORD ITSELF SAYS, "I'M POSSIBLE!"
- SUBCONSCIOUSLY KNOWN -

HEALING CONSIDERATIONS:

LET GO OF THE GARBAGE OF THE PAST

LET GO OF AN OLD IMAGE OF THE PAST

DISCOVER A NEW OUTWARD EXPRESSION OR INWARD ACCEPTANCE

CLEAR BLOCKAGES, DISABLING YOU FROM GAINING VALUE FROM NEW EXPERIENCES

REALISE THAT YOU HAVE VALUE AND IMPACT

MAKE EACH MOMENT COUNT

Notes

_____

_____

_____

_____

_____

_____

_____

_____

_____

B E

M I N D F U L

There are different kinds of people operating in different frequencies in everyday life.

First level of people: having an attitude where they only think of themselves. No thought goes towards everyone else. They only look after themselves. This is based upon survival. Second level of people: where they are totally devoted to a cause, similar to having blind faith in religion. They are so engrossed that they cannot see beyond the walls of their devotion. This relates to the guru and student relationship and many who over-identify with people and organisations, teachers, etc. Third level of people: where they are trying to find their true identity and where they can stretch beyond what they know to become more than they think they are. They can exercise their free will and how they do this is a demonstration of their level of evolution.

Fourth level of people: where they want to be told what to do and be parented. They hand their power and free will to someone to determine their destiny. They want to be taken care of and don't want the responsibility of their own life, often because they don't believe in themselves. This level is very much like being in the armed forces; they are re-programmed and told what to do, and they are looked after.

Fifth level of people: where they are motivated by love and choose to determine their own destiny and create their own opportunities in life. They take responsibility and ownership of the impact of what they do in life.

Exercise: Watch the space between your thoughts. Sit and watch and become aware of a thought, then let go of that thought, and there is a space between that thought and the next thought. Enter the space between thoughts and experience being there for ten minutes without engaging or interacting with it, judging, criticising, analysing, rationalising, intellectualising, or justifying, just being neutral. In this space you step beyond your limited paradigms. Being in the space between is like an eagle flying above the ground looking at its life and things in a neutral, detached manner.

Most exclusively use their intellect to bring about solutions, and these solutions bring more problems than they had before. For extraordinary solutions, you need to access beyond what you know to take you to the next level in life. You do this in the space between. As Einstein stated, "You cannot resolve a problem at the same level of thinking that created it."

Practical exercises addressing BEING MINDFUL:

TO KNOW THE ROAD
AHEAD, ASK THOSE
COMING BACK.
~CHINESE PROVERB -

Exercise 1: Watch for the new opportunities that manifest in your life. Watch the new thoughts and feelings that manifest internally and be aware of the new things that mani-fest externally in your everyday life. This helps to re-calibrate the way your mind functions so you start seeing the new opportunities that manifest in your life.

Exercise 2: Every day write down your new thoughts, feelings, opportunities, and situa-tions that manifest in your everyday life.

Exercise 3: Take note of the levels that you operate on in the different situations and with the different people in your life.

You will encounter the different types of levels as you interact with different people. Slowly, you begin to change some of them and make quality decisions about who you are.

Exercise: everyday write down your new thoughts, feelings, opportunities and situations that manifest in your everyday life.

Exercise: take note of the levels that you operate on, in the different situations and with the different people in your life.

You will encounter the different types of levels as you interact with different people. Slowly, you begin to change some of them and make quality decisions about who you are.

IF A MAN DOES NOT KNOW WHO BREATHES
WITHIN HIM AND IF A MAN DOES NOT KNOW
WHO DREAMS WITHIN HIM;
IT IS NOT BECAUSE THERE IS
ONE SELF WHO ACTS IN THE PHYSICAL UNIVERSE
AND ANOTHER WHO DREAMS AND BREATHES,
IT IS BECAUSE HE HAS BURIED THE
PART OF HIMSELF WHICH BREATHES AND DREAMS.
- UNKNOWN -

CHEETAH - SOUTH AFRICA

REFERENCES:

Lazaris, "Healing the Nature of Health" Recording, www.lazaris.com.

Lazaris, "The Mysterious Power of the Chakras," www.lazaris.com.

Anthony Robbins, "Unlimited Power"

Vladimir Megre, "Anastasia" (Ringing Cedars Press)

CPSIA information can be obtained at www.ICGtesting.com
Printed in the USA
BVIW12n1923030317
477479BV00015B/130